AIDS
& YOU

All About **AIDS**

Books in This Series

AIDS & Politics
AIDS & Poverty
AIDS & Science
AIDS & Society
AIDS & You

AIDS & YOU

C.E. Boberg

AlphaHouse Publishing
New York

All About **AIDS**
AIDS & You

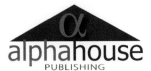

AlphaHouse Publishing
A Division of PEMG Publishing Group, Inc.
201 Harding Avenue
Vestal, New York 13850
www.alphahousepublishing.com

First Printing
9 8 7 6 5 4 3 2 1
ISBN: 978-1-934970-27-0
ISBN (set): 978-1-934970-22-5
   Library of Congress Control Number: 2008930654

Author: Boberg, C.E.

Cover design by Wendy Arakawa.
Interior design by MK Bassett-Harvey.

Printed in India by International Print-O-Pac Limited

 An ISO 9001 Company

Contents

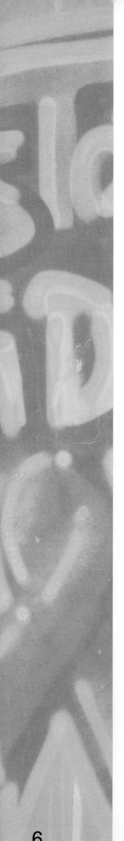

Introduction

What do you know about HIV/AIDS? Where do you get your information? From your friends? From your parents? At school? From television?

You hear a lot about AIDS and HIV these days. But lots of kids—and adults, too—don't really understand HIV/AIDS. They need clearly presented, straightforward facts to replace false information from family and friends and keep themselves safe.

HIV/AIDS is a global epidemic. The facts, from the World Health Organization (WHO) and UNICEF, *can be* scary:

- 33.2 million people were living with HIV/AIDS at the end of 2007.
- 290,000 children under the age of 15 died from HIV/AIDS in 2007.
- More than 2/3 of the population of sub-Saharan Africa is infected with HIV/AIDS.
- Over 15 million children under the age of 18 have lost one or both parents to AIDS, and millions more have been made vulnerable.

No matter how scary the facts seem, they should not overpower us. The world is fighting HIV/AIDS every day at the global and the individual level. There is no cure for

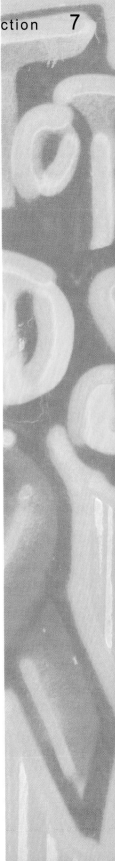

HIV, but there are treatments. However, many people in the world continue to go without the treatments they need. In fact, the Joint United Nations Programme on HIV/AIDS (UNAIDS) reports that, globally, less than one person in five at risk of HIV has access to basic HIV prevention services and only 31% of people who needed HIV treatment had access to it by the end of 2007. This series talks about why, and what organizations such as the WHO and UNAIDS are doing about the problem.

These books discuss the effects of different aspects of society on the HIV/AIDS pandemic. For example, gender, age, poverty, political struggles, and geography all affect peoples' overall health and access to treatment. In addition, many people, afraid of the social stigma and perceived death sentence of an HIV diagnosis, avoid seeking help when it is needed.

The truth is vital to preventing further spread of the disease. People need to get tested, learn their status, and begin antiretroviral therapy treatment in order to help prevent spreading the disease to others. Education is key to this process of prevention. This series promotes prevention and action through education. The books are intended for distribution to families, libraries, and schools around the world to help reduce fear, increase knowledge, and promote prevention.

The series also touches on what the world is doing to end the HIV/AIDS epidemic and offers suggestions for how readers can get involved at the individual, community, or global level.

Here's what you need to know

- HIV stands for Human Immune Deficiency Virus. It's the virus that causes AIDS.
- AIDS stands for Acquired Immunodeficiency Syndrome.
- HIV/AIDS hurts your body's ability to fight off other diseases and infections.
- You CAN'T catch HIV/AIDS from touching an infected person or being around an infected person.
- The only way to catch HIV/AIDS is from an infected person's body fluids.
- You can be infected:
  - during sex.
  - by sharing dirty drug, tattoo, or piercing needles.
  - via mother-to-infant transmission.
- In the 1970s and 1980s, people caught HIV/AIDS from blood transfusions, but now blood donors are screened before they can give blood.
- Although scientists have not found a cure for HIV/AIDS, they have found better medicines that help a person with the virus live longer, with fewer symptoms.
- Scientists are still looking for either a cure or a vaccine that would keep people from getting the disease.
- HIV medicines are very expensive and not everyone can afford them.
- Poverty and HIV/AIDS are two of the biggest problems facing the world today—and they are connected to each other.

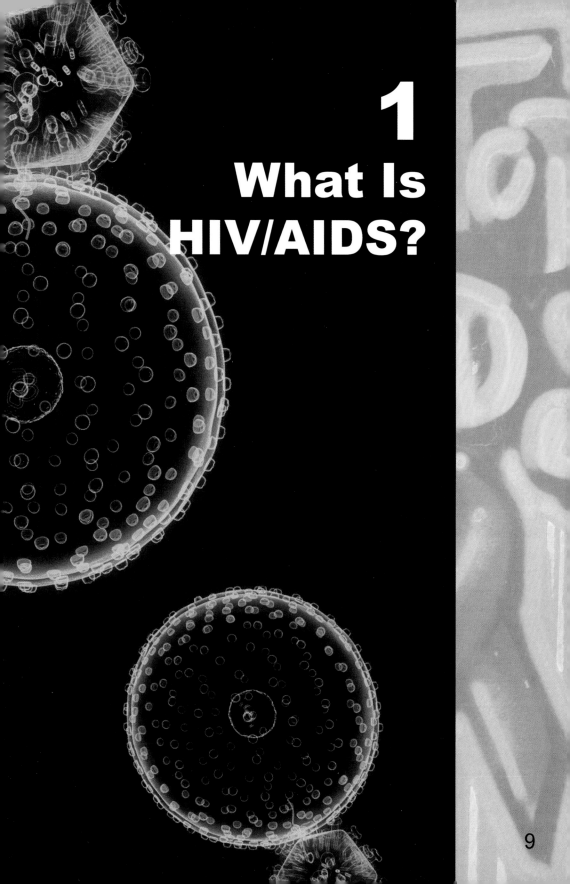

1
What Is
HIV/AIDS?

Words to Understand

If something is *acquired*, you get it through something you do (rather than it coming to you through your genes or some other part of your make-up over which you have no control).

Your *immune system* fights off germs and keeps you from getting sick.

A *deficiency* is when you don't have enough of something.

A *syndrome* is a collection of disease symptoms doctors don't completely understand.

Antibodies are special proteins in your blood that fight germs.

If something is *infectious* it can pass from one person to another.

Transfusions are injections of blood or blood components into the bloodstream.

Developed nations are countries where the majority of the population have higher incomes with all the services they need. There are many industries in these countries. Most of Japan, the United States, Canada, Israel, and many of the countries in Europe are all developed countries.

Developing nations are countries where most of the people live in poverty and have few educational, professional, and medical opportunities. Much of the population usually depends on farming for their livelihoods, and there are few industries. Most of the countries of Africa and South America are considered to be developing nations.

Crises are turning points in life. Often the outcomes of these moments are terrible—but the potential for new growth and a better world is also present in every crisis as well.

You hear a lot about AIDS and HIV these days. You've probably seen television shows and movies where characters had this disease. You hear about it at school. You may even know someone who has it. You may think it's connected somehow to homosexuals. But lots of kids—and adults too—don't really understand what HIV/AIDS is. They don't know how you catch it, who gets it, or what causes it. Lots of people don't even know what these letters stand for.

HIV stands for human immunodeficiency virus. It's the virus that causes AIDS—acquired immunodeficiency syndrome. People may have the HIV virus in their bodies, and still have no symptoms that they're sick. As the disease becomes worse, though, and people develop symptoms, it often is referred to as AIDS.

Acquired immunodeficiency syndrome—AIDS—got its name because:

- It is **acquired**; in other words, it is a condition that has to be passed to you from another person. It cannot be inherited from your parents or passed along to you by your genes. This means if your boyfriend has HIV/AIDS you could catch it from him—but if your grandmother who lives in another country has HIV/AIDS, you're not going to discover that she passed it on to you.

- It affects the body's *immune* system, the part of the body that fights off diseases.
- It is considered a *deficiency* because it makes the immune system stop working the way it should.
- At first doctors thought it was a *syndrome* because people with AIDS experience a number of different symptoms and diseases. A syndrome is a word doctors use for a collection of symptoms they don't completely understand, and when the term AIDS was first used, doctors only knew about the disease's late stages. They didn't understand exactly what was making people sick. Today, doctors think that "HIV disease" is a better name, but AIDS is still the name that most people use.

Your Immune System

The worst thing about AIDS is that it hurts your immune system—the special cells in your blood that fight off germs

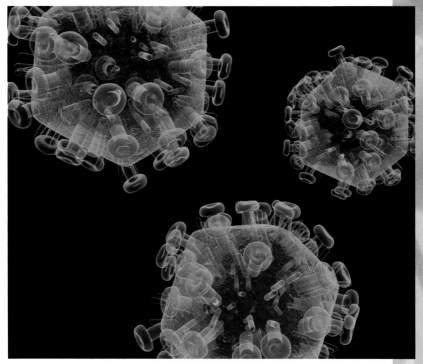

The HIV virus is a tiny organism that needs a host cell in order to act like a living thing. Unlike most living things, viruses have no cells. Instead, they are made mostly of genetic material that changes the cells they infect.

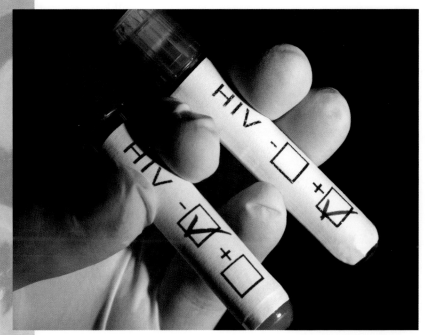

If you think you may have been exposed to the HIV virus, go to your doctor or clinic and get your blood tested. It may be scary to find out the truth—but it's better to know. Even if the news isn't good, new treatments mean that a person with HIV may often live a healthy life for a long time.

and keep you from getting sick. When this happens, you can get sick with other infections, and your body won't be able to fight off the illness. People with AIDS often actually die from another disease (such as an infection caused by a fungus, pneumonia, brain infections, or cancer).

When a virus or bacteria (what we often call germs) get into your body through a cut, through the air you breathe, or through something you've eaten, special cells in your blood, white blood cells called helper T cells, also called CD4 lymphocytes, get busy. They pass along the message to another group of white blood cells—B cells—telling them to make the weapons (called **antibodies**) they need to kill the germs. If a virus or bacteria makes its way past the antibodies, it can cause an infection. When that happens, a different type of T cell recognizes the change in the infected cell and kills it. This prevents the infection from spreading. At least this is what is *supposed* to happen.

When someone has HIV, eventually, she will no longer be able to fight off infections that other people have no problem resisting. As HIV grows within her body, her

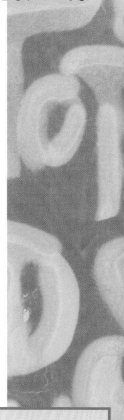

immune system gets weaker and weaker. She will become more ill more often, especially with certain kinds of cancer and pneumonia.

Doctors say that a person has AIDS when:

- he has tested positive for HIV in his blood.
- he has had one or more AIDS-related infections or illnesses.
- the number of CD4 lymphocytes has reached or fallen below 200 per cubic millimeter of blood (a healthy person's T-cell count ranges between 450 and 1,200).

A few people will have AIDS within a few months from the time they are first exposed to HIV, but that's not usual. In most people, symptoms do not show up for ten to twelve years. It's very important to find out if a person has HIV as soon as possible, because doctors now

The Spread of HIV/AIDS

This table shows how many people were living with AIDS in different parts of the world in 2004, compared to 3 years earlier.

Region	2001	2004
Sub-Sahara Africa	23.8 million	25.4 million
South & Southeast Asia	5.9 million	6.4 million
Latin American	1.4 million	1.7 million
Eastern & Central Europe	890,000	1.4 million
East Asia & Pacific	680,000	1.1 million
North America	950,000	1 million
Western Europe	540,000	610,000
North Africa & Middle East	340,000	540,000
Caribbean	400,000	440,000
Oceania	24,000	35,000

In the years since 2004, the numbers have continued to climb.

have medicines that can make most people go even longer before developing AIDS.

The one to three months after a person is first infected with the HIV virus is when that person is most *infectious*. The amount of virus in her system is at its highest and T-cell counts are at their lowest, which means she is most likely to pass along the disease to others. During this time, her body has not had time to react to the virus and produce the cells that will fight the virus. Meanwhile, the virus is reproducing itself within the body.

You can't tell that all this is happening. On the outside, there are no symptoms, and a person who is infected can look and feel perfectly well for many years; he may not even know he is infected. As the immune system gets weaker, however, the person becomes more likely to catch the illnesses that the immune system would normally have been able to fight. As time goes by, he is more likely to become ill more often and develop AIDS.

How Does HIV Spread?

First, how does it not spread? HIV CANNOT be spread by:

- shaking hands with someone who has HIV/AIDS
- hugging someone who has HIV/AIDS

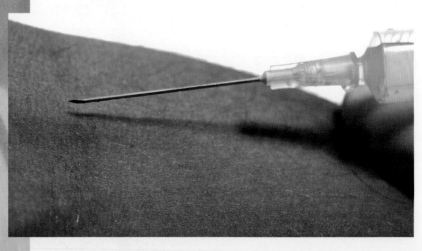

Real People

Ryan White began 1984 as a typical thirteen-year-old. He had hemophilia, but it was being treated. He went to school and had friends, just like most kids his age. Then Ryan and his family found out he had caught HIV through the blood products he had received to treat his hemophilia. The HIV had already advanced to AIDS. Doctors told Ryan and his family that he only had six months to live.

Ryan wanted to spend the last months of his life doing what he had been doing, going to school and being with friends. But the school didn't want him there. People were afraid Ryan's illness might "rub off" on the other students. Ryan's battle to be allowed to attend school made news first in the United States and then all over the world. Because of Ryan, people all over the world started thinking about AIDS.

On April 8, 1990, Ryan White lost his battle with AIDS. He was only nineteen when he died, but he had done a lot with his life. Because he fought hard to make people realize that AIDS is a problem we must all face, laws were passed to help people with HIV/AIDS, television shows were made, magazine articles were written, and education programs were started in schools. The world began to work together to fight this terrible disease—all because one young boy was brave enough to take a stand.

- sharing eating utensils with someone who has HIV/AIDS
- being in the same room with someone who has HIV/AIDS
- touching something that someone with HIV/AIDS has touched
- breathing the same air as someone with HIV/AIDS

Researchers are developing new medicines that are more effective at fighting the HIV virus. Unfortunately, some of the areas of the world that need this medication most are too poor to afford it.

Doctors have never found any cases where someone caught HIV by doing any of these things with a family member, friend, or coworker.

The ONLY way to become infected with HIV is through certain body fluids. The person infected with the virus carries it in blood, semen, vaginal secretions, and breast milk. In order for you to catch HIV, one of these fluids from a person with HIV would have to enter your

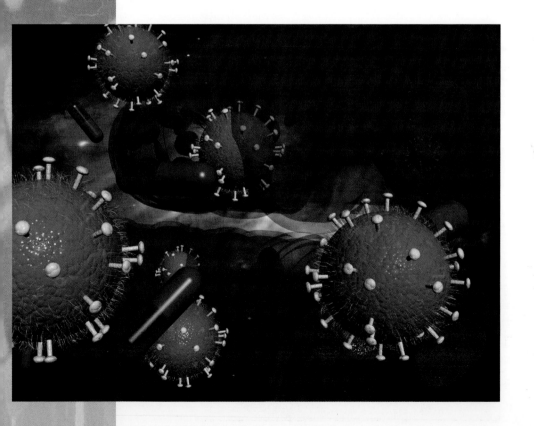

bloodstream. Here are the most common ways that HIV could get into your blood:

- during unprotected sex (sex where no condom is used)
- during the kind of drug use where the user "shoots up" with a needle (if the needle is dirty and was used by someone who has HIV)
- through a cut or sore on the skin.

The most common way to catch HIV is through unprotected sexual intercourse. This means any kind of sex—oral, anal, or vaginal. Women are more at risk for catching HIV this way than are their male partners, but women can also pass along HIV to men through sexual intercourse.

Some drug users share needles and other equipment. This makes intravenous drug users another group of people who often get HIV. Needles used for body piercing and tattooing can also carry HIV and should not be reused. If you decide to get a piercing or a tattoo, be sure to only have it done by someone who uses only clean equipment.

The youngest people with AIDS—the babies—generally get the disease from their mothers. In most of these cases, the mother does not know she is infected, especially since there can be many years between when she was exposed to the virus and when she first gets symptoms. If there is any chance a woman has been exposed to HIV, she should be tested for the virus before becoming pregnant. Medicine can be given to pregnant women with HIV to

Global Statistics on HIV/AIDS

Number of people living with HIV

Adults	38.0 million
Women	17.5 million
Children under age 15	2.3 million
Total	40.3 million

People Newly Infected with HIV
(according to UN and WHO research)

Adults	4.2 million
Children under age 15	700,000
Total	4.9 million

AIDS Deaths

Adults	2.6 million
Children under age 15	570,000
Total	3.1 million

Did You Know?

The virus that causes AIDS changes quickly. This means that today's medicines may not be able to fight the new strains of HIV.

protect to their babies during pregnancy. After the baby is born, women with HIV should not breastfeed, so that the virus isn't passed to their babies through breast milk.

HIV/AIDS and Blood Transfusions

In the 1970s and early 1980s, before anyone knew very much about HIV/AIDS, blood donors who didn't know they had the disease gave their blood to hospitals and at Red Cross blood drives—and the virus got into the blood supply that was given out to sick or injured people who needed blood *transfusions*. Eventually, doctors realized that some people were catching HIV/AIDS from blood transfusions. Beginning in 1985, the blood supply has been tested for HIV, and there is no longer much risk that someone will get HIV/AIDS from a blood transfusion. However, people who received transfusions between 1975 and 1985 had a high risk of receiving infected blood. Among those most at risk were people with hemophilia.

Hemophilia

Hemophilia is an illness in which blood clots much more slowly than normal. As a result, small cuts and other injuries can cause heavy bleeding. Boys are more apt to have this disease than girls.

People with hemophilia must use blood and blood products to control bleeding episodes. This made them vulnerable to the contaminated blood supply between 1975 and 1985. Some reports indicate that during this time as many as half of the individuals with hemophilia were infected with HIV through blood and blood products. According to the Web site www.hivpositive.com, an estimated 10,000 people with hemophilia have HIV today.

You cannot get HIV by donating blood. And today, the risk of becoming infected with

Using a condom is one of the best ways to protect yourself against the HIV virus.

HIV through the use of blood and blood products is greatly reduced for individuals with hemophilia. More careful screening of blood donors has been one reason for this; blood from every donor is checked for HIV before it is used. New methods of treating the blood and blood products, including the use of heat, have also reduced the risk.

Treatment for HIV/AIDS

Up until recently, if you found out you had HIV, you thought you would die soon. Today, however, some people who have the virus have still not developed AIDS even after many years. AIDS has no cure yet, but many people with HIV are living longer and staying healthier. New medicines have made this possible.

HIV does not respond well to just one single medicine. Instead, doctors have found that the disease responds best to a combination of various medicines. Taking so many pills can be hard to remember —and it's expensive.

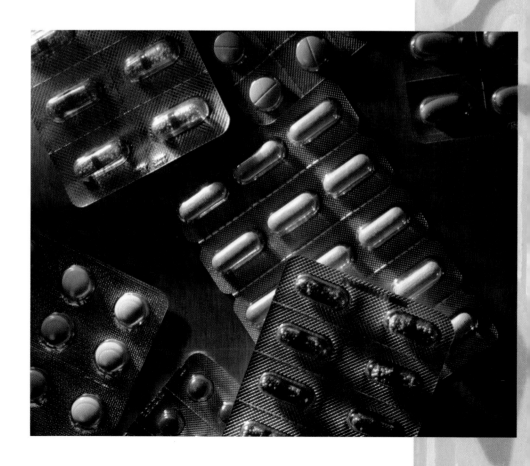

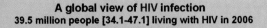

A global view of HIV infection
39.5 million people [34.1-47.1] living with HIV in 2006

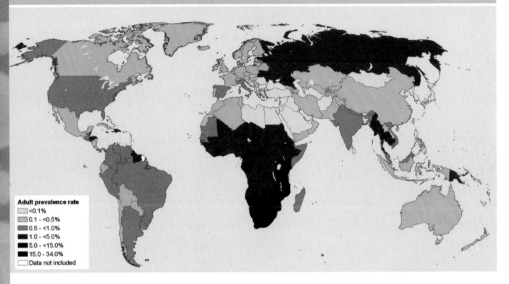

Adult prevalence rate
- <0.1%
- 0.1 - <0.5%
- 0.5 - <1.0%
- 1.0 - <5.0%
- 5.0 - <15.0%
- 15.0 - 34.0%
- Data not included

The boundaries and names shown and the designations used on this map do not imply the expression of any opinion whatsoever on the part of the World Health Organization concerning the legal status of any country, territory, city or area or of its authorities, or concerning the delimitation of its frontiers or boundaries. Dotted lines on maps represent approximate border lines for which there may not yet be full agreement.

Data Source: WHO / UNAIDS
Map Production: Public Health Mapping and GIS
Communicable Diseases (CDS)
World Health Organization

 World Health Organization

© WHO 2007. All rights reserved

For many people living with HIV/AIDS, a single medicine does not work. Most take a combination of many drugs, sometimes called a "cocktail." The medicines have to be taken a certain way at certain times in order for them to work. They work together to reduce the level of HIV in the body, allowing the body's own CD4 lymphocytes to return to healthier levels. This is good news. But it doesn't mean that HIV/AIDS is no longer a huge problem in our world today.

For one thing, some people have a hard time remembering when and how to take so many different kinds of medicines. Imagine if you had to take four or more different pills every day at different times throughout the day. You'd probably forget sometimes. So do lots of people who are taking these medicines. But when they do, the medicines don't work as well for them, and new forms of the virus can develop.

The medicines also have some bad side effects. They can damage a person's kidneys, heart, and bones. If this happens, the person cannot keep taking the medicines.

But the worst problem with these medicines is that they are very expensive. Around the world, many of the people living with HIV/AIDS are also living in poverty. They may have no money to buy the medicine or even go to the doctor. They may live in a region so poor that they don't even have a doctor or clinic nearby where they could go if they did have money.

People living with HIV/AIDS in North America, Europe, and other **developed nations** have a better chance of living longer, even when they are poor. Many of these countries have special programs to help bring AIDS medicines to people living in poverty. These programs are not perfect; many times people may make just enough money that they don't qualify, but not enough money that they can afford to buy the medicines on their own. But

These hands belong to poor children in Ethiopia. Their risk of contracting HIV is high, and poverty makes their situation worse.

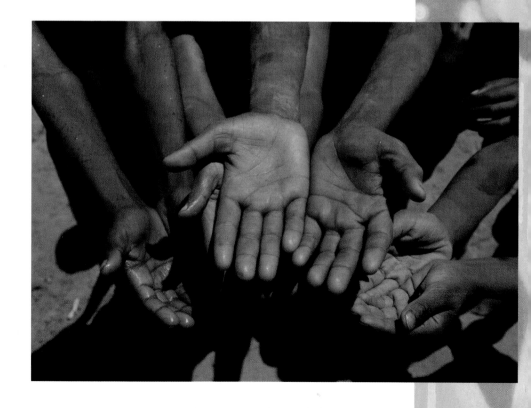

How Can You Keep Yourself Safe?

The only way to be sure you won't catch HIV/AIDS is to protect yourself from other people's body fluids. Sex is the way most people come into contact with body fluids. So if you don't want to catch HIV/AIDS, you need to protect yourself by not having sex until you are sure it is safe. Women and men don't need to worry about getting HIV/AIDS from each other:

- if neither partner ever had sex with anyone else.

- if neither partner ever shared needles.

- if neither partner currently has or ever had HIV/AIDS.

What Is Safer Sex?

The only way to be absolutely certain you don't catch something from a sexual partner is to not have sex until you know you're in safe relationship where both of you will keep your promises to be faithful to each other. However, "safer sex" is anything you can do to lower your risk of getting HIV/AIDS (or another disease) if you do choose to have sex outside a safe relationship. The most important ways to reduce your risk are:

- Keep your partner's body fluids out of your body, including your vagina, anus, or mouth. The body fluids to be most careful about are blood, semen, vaginal fluids, and the runny discharge from sores.

Safer sex also means protecting your partner:

- Don't allow your body fluids to get into your partner's body.

- Don't have sex if you have sores or other symptoms of infection.

- Have routine checkups for sexually transmitted infections.

- Get the correct treatment if you become infected.

When you are a child, it's the job of the adults in your life to protect you and keep you safe. As you get older, though, it will be up to you to protect yourself from danger. Take care of yourself! Make sure you're not one of the millions of people around the world who are living with HIV/AIDS.

An AIDS Vaccine?

Less than a hundred years ago, many people died from diseases like small pox and polio. When researchers created a shot—a vaccine—that keeps people from catching these diseases, they saved millions of lives. One day, scientists hope to discovers a vaccine that will protect against HIV/AIDS in the same way.

as researchers find new ways to treat HIV/AIDS, these people may one day have access to better medicine and even a vaccine.

Some of the world's *developing nations* don't have even the most basic medicines to treat their people, let alone the medications that treat HIV/AIDS. Sometimes the nation's government controls the medicines, and the government decides who gets the medicine, often based on how much money the person has. The big companies that make the medicines are also part of the problem. Sometimes these companies have refused to sell drugs at lower prices to the developing world.

Poverty and AIDS are enormous crises in today's world, both in developed and developing countries. You can't separate them from each other—poverty makes AIDS a bigger problem, and AIDS makes poverty a bigger problem. We have to understand each side of the problem—and we have to fight them both.

Ask the Doctor

Q: My boyfriend and I are careful when we have sex. He always makes sure he pulls out before he comes. My older sister says I can't get pregnant if he does this. Does it also mean I wouldn't catch AIDS from him if he had it?

No! This is not a safe way to protect yourself against either pregnancy or a sexually transmitted disease like HIV/AIDS. During sexual intercourse, a man's penis has a little bit of semen on it even before he ejaculates (or "comes"). Although this is a very small amount, it is enough that you could possibly become pregnant—or get HIV/AIDS from him if he is infected. Latex condoms are the only birth-control method that can also help protect you from HIV/AIDS and other infections. And remember—use condoms correctly with water-based lubricants, to reduce the chance that they could break.

STRAIGHT FROM THE SOURCE

(From the 2004 World Health Organization (WHO) document Protecting Young People from HIV and AIDS.)

Measures to reduce the vulnerability of young people and to reduce risk are complementary and part of a continuum. In terms of the sexual transmission of HIV this is well expressed as:

❑ DELAY—your first sexual experience,

❑ REDUCE—the number of your sexual partners,

❑ PROTECT—yourself and your partner by using a condom.

This approach encourages those who are at no or low risk to remain safe, and encourages all others to move in the direction of greater safety. It helps to create a climate where adolescents can more easily delay the onset of sexual experience, which is the only 100% effective way of avoiding HIV. It addresses the need to reduce the number of sexual partners, since risks rise rapidly with multiple partners. It emphasizes the need for consistent and correct use of condoms. Without condoms, those young people who do not succeed in abstaining are left unprotected at very high risk, and there would be little prospect of reducing HIV levels in the community. Millions of young people would be left to their fate, including girls who are powerless to abstain because sex is forced or coerced. Promoting abstinence and promoting condoms are not alternatives—but complementary parts of an effective approach. Condom use is promoted in order to protect those who are having sex, not to undermine those who are not.

What Do You Think?

- According to this WHO document, what is the only 100 percent effective way to avoid HIV?

- Why do you think the chances of getting HIV go up the more times you have sex with a different person?

- Why do you think some people object to teaching kids about how to use condoms?

- Why do you think other people object to only teaching kids about "abstinence" (not having sex at all)?

- What approach is WHO recommending in this document regarding the condom-abstinence question?

Find Out More

To find out more about HIV/AIDS check out these Web sites:

The AIDS Handbook: Written for Middle School Kids by Middle School Kids
www.eastchester.k12.ny.us/schools/ms/AIDS/AIDS1.html

Let's Talk: Children, Families, and HIV
www.kidstalkaids.org/education/index.html

YouthAIDS (What You Can Do to Change the World)
www.youthaids.org

Words to Understand

Blood products are different parts of blood that are separated out and given to people who only need one part of the blood. Blood is made out of plasma, red blood cells, platelets, and clotting agents.

An epidemic is the outbreak of a disease that affects an unexpectedly large number of a population.

Hepatitis C is a virus that affects the liver, leading to infections and liver damage. IV drug users with HIV often also have Hepatitis C, also known as HCV.

Intravenous, or IV, injections or lines are used to get drugs directly into the veins. They are used in hospitals to give fluid and medication to patients; drug users also use them to inject heroin or other street drugs.

A lesion can be either a normal cut or a sore that comes from an infection.

Mucous membranes line parts of the body that lead from the inside to the outside, like the intestines and the lungs. Outer mucous membranes have pink, moist skin, and include the lips, eyelids, and genitals.

During pregnancy, women and their babies are given prenatal (before birth) care that often includes vitamins, a healthy diet, and frequent medical check-ups.

HIV is a retrovirus, a type of virus with a fatty protective coating on the outside and viral copying material on the inside. Patients with HIV are given antiretroviral drugs to slow the change from HIV to AIDS.

Here's what you need to know

- You CAN'T catch HIV/AIDS from touching an infected person or being around an infected person.
- The only way to catch HIV/AIDS is from an infected person's body fluids.
- Health care workers are often exposed to HIV-positive blood, but hospitals have special practices set up to keep their employees safe.
- HIV can be passed on during childbirth if the mother has not received good prenatal care.

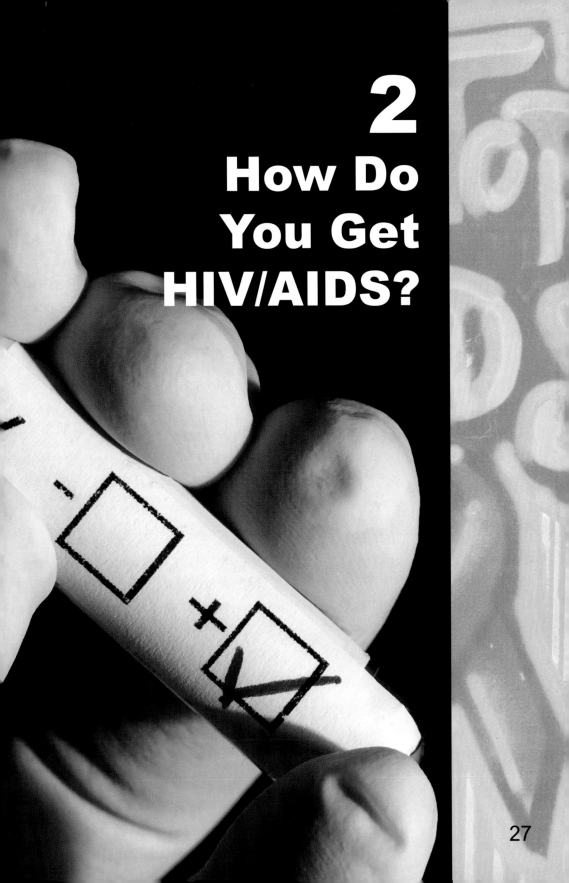

2
How Do You Get HIV/AIDS?

The more informed you are about the ways that HIV is transmitted, the more you can understand how to protect yourself while still respecting people who have HIV/AIDS. One of the most important ways to understand the spread of HIV/AIDS is to know the ways that it can't be spread.

How HIV Is NOT Spread

Here are some myths about how HIV/AIDS is spread:

You can get AIDS from shaking hands with, hugging, or even being in the same room as a person who has HIV/AIDS.

No! Some people might think that they can get HIV this way because they think it spreads through the air, but this is absolutely not true. HIV/AIDS is spread through direct

You cannot get AIDS by shaking hands with an infected person; AIDS can only be transmitted through the exchange of certain body fluids, like blood, semen, and breast milk.

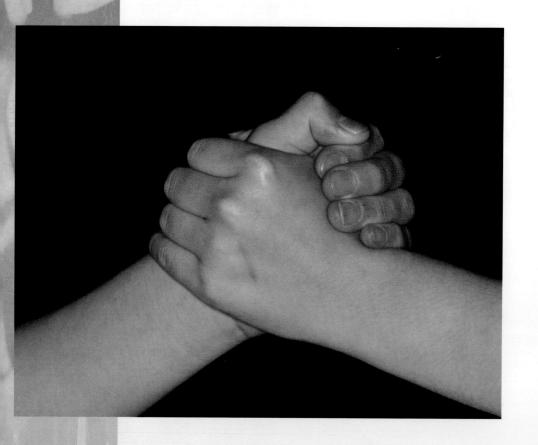

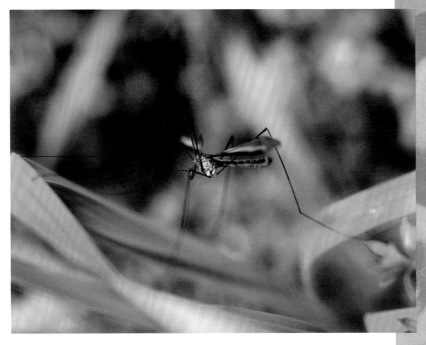

You cannot get AIDS from a mosquito bite, as a mosquito does not actually inject blood into you. Also, the HIV virus cannot reproduce in insects, making it impossible to get HIV this way.

blood or sexual contact with an infected person. It is possible to be physically close to an infected person without ever exposing yourself to HIV/AIDS.

You can get AIDS from sharing a fork or cup with a person who has HIV/AIDS.
No! Although saliva is a bodily fluid, HIV is present in it in such tiny amounts that it is impossible to spread in this way. Sweat, tears, and saliva are all fluids that cannot spread HIV.

You can get AIDS from being bitten by a mosquito that has bitten a person who has HIV/AIDS.
No! When a mosquito bites you, the blood that it has taken from other people never leaves its body. Also, the virus does not reproduce in insects – it only lives for a very short time inside the mosquito's body before dying. There is no risk of contracting HIV/AIDS from a mosquito bite.

Doctors have never found any cases where someone caught HIV from a family member, friend, or coworker just by being close to them. You can treat a friend with HIV/AIDS the same way that you treat any of your friends. Sometimes people will be cruel to a person with HIV/AIDS because they are afraid and don't understand that they are safe. This is not just hurtful to the person with HIV/AIDS; it's also hurtful to the person who is afraid because it shows that they don't know enough about HIV/AIDS to protect themselves correctly.

How HIV Is Spread

The ONLY way to become infected with HIV is to come into contact with certain bodily fluids. The person infected with the virus carries it in blood, semen, vaginal secretions, and breast milk. Small amounts of the virus are present in saliva and tears, but there has never been a case of HIV being transmitted through either of these fluids. In order for you to catch HIV, one of these fluids from a person with HIV would have to enter your bloodstream.

Sexual Activity

The most common way to catch HIV is through unprotected sexual intercourse. This means any kind of sex, not just sex between two homosexuals. However, unprotected anal sex is more likely than vaginal sex to transmit HIV to the uninfected partner not only because the anus is lined with tissue that is much more fragile than vaginal tissue, but also because it does not have a natural lubricating system like the vagina does. Both of these factors can lead to small tears where the virus can travel into the bloodstream. Both heterosexual and homosexual partners are at risk for HIV exposure if they have unprotected anal sex.

It is a common misunderstanding that women are not likely to contract HIV, but they are actually more at risk for catching HIV during vaginal intercourse than are their male partners. Since the vagina is a *mucous membrane,* it has a direct connection with the bloodstream and can pass the virus from the skin to the blood. Women can also pass along HIV to men, but it is less common than male-to-female transmission.

There is also a small chance that HIV can be transmitted through oral sex. Although very few cases of this type have been reported, it is possible to spread the virus in this way if the partner who is giving oral sex has any cuts in his or her mouth. The risk goes up if this person also has an STI, has recently brushed or flossed his teeth (which can lead to bleeding gums), or has a canker sore or other type of oral *lesion*. The person receiving oral sex has a relatively low risk of getting HIV if their partner is infected, because saliva does not carry enough of the virus to pose a risk of infection.

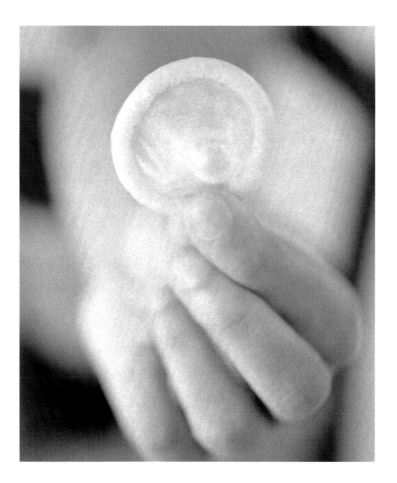

Ask the Doctor

Q: My friend has sex with a lot of different girls. He never uses condoms, but he always makes sure the girls he has sex with take birth control. He says that since he's not gay, he can't get AIDS. Is this true?

No! Actually, he can't get AIDS from having unprotected sex, but he can get HIV, which causes AIDS. A lot of people used to think that HIV/AIDS was a gay disease because it first appeared in the gay community, but heterosexual people get HIV too. Your friend isn't just at risk for catching HIV—he could also contract syphilis, gonorrhea, or herpes from unprotected sex with multiple partners. He should get tested for STDs and read up on safer sex practices. If he doesn't wear condoms because they don't fit or he has a latex allergy, he should look into alternatives like the female condom or polyurethane condoms.

In any type of sexual activity, the risk of transmitting HIV is increased if either partner is intoxicated, has an STI, or has any open sores. Intoxication from any type of drug or alcohol is risky because it can lead to blackouts, poor decision-making, or mistakes like unwanted or unprotected sex. STIs and open sores increase the risk of transmitting HIV because at the site of infection the skin is usually swollen or broken, providing direct access to the bloodstream. STIs also increase the risk because the immune system sends large numbers of CD4 cells, the same cells that HIV affects, to fight infections at their source. If the person is exposed to HIV while they have an STI, it is more likely that their CD4 cells will be infected and they will contract HIV. **Safer sex** dramatically decreases the risk of HIV transmission, but remember that it is safer sex, not safe sex! Remember to use your judgment when engaging in sexual activity to reduce your risk even further.

One type of sexual activity that cannot transmit HIV is masturbation. If you are HIV negative and you pleasure yourself, there is no way that your body can generate HIV in response. There are several ways that you can engage in sexual activity without risking HIV exposure: masturbation, mutual masturbation, kissing, hugging, or petting.

Intravenous Drug Use

Drug users are also more at-risk for HIV infection than most people, especially if they reuse or share needles and equipment. Every time someone injects a drug into his veins, whether it is heroin or a legal drug to treat an illness, he must pull up on the plunger of the syringe to check for blood, which confirms that he has inserted the needle into the vein. Some of the blood gets into the syringe, and it will stay in the tip even after completing the injection. HIV does not live for very long outside of the body because it dries up and falls apart, but when the blood gets stuck in the tip of a syringe, it is unable to dry up and can stay active. If another person uses the same syringe, she will inject the leftover blood into her body, which can easily infect her with HIV. Some countries have set up needle-exchange programs to cut down on the amount of HIV infections among drug users. In these programs, drug users can bring in their used hypodermic needles and get new needles, sterilization equipment, and HIV tests, often free of charge.

The HIV virus can live in the tips of used needles for more than a month; this means that it is very important that drug users use clean needles in order to protect themselves from getting sick.

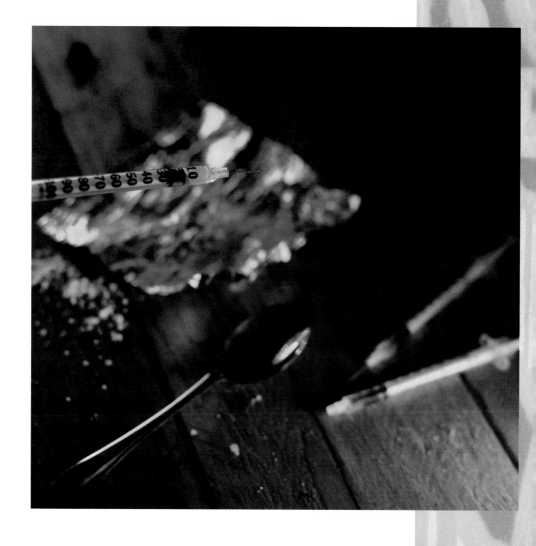

Real People

Keith was a senior in high school when he was diagnosed with HIV. He organized a blood drive with other seniors to fulfill his community service requirement, but he didn't intend to give blood. After fighting with his girlfriend about it, he finally caved in and gave blood. A few weeks later, he got a call from the program that held the blood drive and was told that he needed to make an appointment.

He was HIV-positive. A sexual encounter with a man had exposed him to the virus, but he had thought that, since he wasn't gay or promiscuous, he couldn't be at risk. After Keith's diagnosis, he thought about all of the things that he had planned to do with his life that now seemed out of reach—but a little voice in his mind told him that everything would be okay.

Twelve years later, he is okay: Keith is thirty and healthy, an HIV writer and educator for thebody.com, a comprehensive website devoted to HIV/AIDS.

(From "What's Goin' On? The Little Voice Within," August 2006)

Piercing and Tattooing

Needles used for body piercing and tattooing can also carry HIV and should not be reused. If you decide to get a piercing or a tattoo, be sure to have it done by a doctor or a piercer who wears surgical gloves and sterilizes his equipment. Although there has not been a documented case of a person getting HIV from a piercing or tattoo, *Hepatitis C* and other blood-borne diseases have been transmitted in this way. Also, during the healing process of a piercing or tattoo, the wound is more at risk of infection by both HIV and treatable bacterial infections and should not be exposed to any type of bodily fluids.

Other Nonsexual Sources of HIV Infection

Doctors and nurses are another group of people who have a higher risk of exposure to HIV, simply because of their contact with bodily fluids. However, the Centers for Disease Control in the US has implemented a set of *universal precautions* that greatly lowers the chance of coming into contact with HIV-infected fluid. The rate of hospital-related HIV exposure is fairly low, and there are special HIV-prevention procedures for people who are involved in needle-stick accidents.

Tattoos are another risk factor for AIDS. If you are thinking about getting a tattoo, make sure the artist uses new, sterilized needles and that he wears gloves.

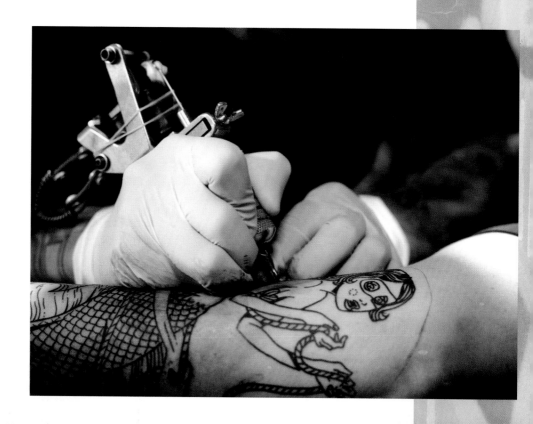

Before 1985, when AIDS was still a new and relatively unknown disease, hospitals didn't have a way to test for HIV in donated blood. As a result, a large number of people who received blood transfusions also developed HIV/AIDS. Many of these people were hemophiliacs, people whose blood is unable to clot when they get a cut, who got transfusions of blood or **blood products**. Even though this was a widespread problem when the AIDS *epidemic* first started, there has been very little risk of HIV transmission through the use of blood products since 1985, when tests for HIV were first developed and used on the blood supply.

While medication can prevent mothers from passing HIV to their babies during pregnancy, there is some risk of transmission during childbirth. Because of this, often mothers with HIV should give birth via caesarean section in order to minimize the chance of passing the virus on to the child.

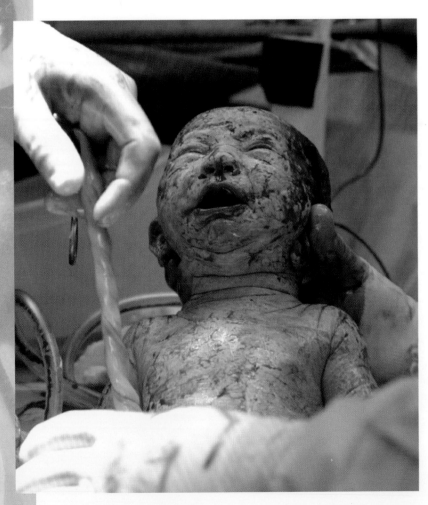

The last common infection path of HIV/AIDS is through childbirth, when HIV is passed from a mother to her baby. The mother often doesn't know she is infected, especially since there can be many years between the time she was exposed to the virus and when she would first show any symptoms. If there is any chance a woman has been exposed to HIV, she should be tested for the virus before becoming pregnant. It is possible for an HIV-positive woman to have a healthy baby, although she must take certain medications and precautions in order to keep her baby from contracting the virus. If the mother has received proper *prenatal* care and delivers safely, there is only a 2% risk that her baby will contract HIV during childbirth. However, if the mother has not been on *antiretroviral* drugs during her pregnancy, she should give birth via caesarean section in order to minimize the risk of passing on HIV during birth. After the baby is born, women with HIV are often advised not to breastfeed so that the virus isn't passed to their babies through breast milk. However, in developing countries this may not be an option.

STRAIGHT FROM THE SOURCE

(From the CDC's website, address: www.cdc.gov/hiv/ resources/qa/qa35.htm)

How well does HIV survive outside the body?

Scientists and medical authorities agree that HIV does not survive well outside the body, making the possibility of environmental transmission remote. HIV is found in varying concentrations or amounts in blood, semen, vaginal fluid, breast milk, saliva, and tears. To obtain data on the survival of HIV, laboratory studies have required the use of artificially high concentrations of laboratory-grown virus. Although these unnatural concentrations of HIV can be kept alive for days or even weeks under precisely controlled and limited laboratory conditions, CDC studies have shown that drying of even these high concentrations of HIV reduces the amount of infectious virus by 90 to 99 percent within several hours. Since the HIV concentrations used in laboratory studies are much higher than those actually found in blood or other specimens, drying of HIV-infected human blood or other body fluids reduces the theoretical risk of environmental transmission to that which has been observed—essentially zero. Incorrect interpretations of conclusions drawn from laboratory studies have in some instances caused unnecessary alarm.

Results from laboratory studies should not be used to assess specific personal risk of infection because (1) the amount of virus studied is not found in human specimens or elsewhere in nature, and (2) no one has been identified as infected with HIV due to contact with an environmental surface. Additionally, HIV is unable to reproduce outside its living host (unlike many bacteria or fungi, which may do so under suitable conditions), except under laboratory conditions; therefore, it does not spread or maintain infectiousness outside its host.

What Do You Think?

- According to this CDC document, does HIV multiply outside of the human body?

- Why do you think it is not possible for a person to contract HIV from casual contact?

- If the concentrations of HIV used in laboratory tests are much higher than those that occur in human blood, do you think that HIV in humans dies slower or faster than laboratory-created HIV once it starts drying up? Why?

- What are the similarities and differences between HIV and bacteria or fungi?

- What does the CDC suggest about measuring risk of HIV transmission based on laboratory studies?

Find Out More

To find out more about the transmission of HIV, check out these Web sites:

The CDC's basic guide to HIV:
www.cdc.gov/hiv/topics/basic/index.htm

Information on transmission of HIV:
www.hiv.com/page7.html

Basic facts about HIV/AIDS from amfAR:
www.amfar.org/cgi-bin/iowa/abouthiv/index.html

Here's what you need to know

- There are over 30 million people living with HIV/AIDS in the world.
- Over 2 million of those people are children, and still more are teenagers and young adults.
- HIV does not discriminate because of race, gender, sexual preference, or age.
- Young people became involved in many AIDS support organizations in the beginning of the AIDS crisis in the United States.
- Teens are less aware of the risks of HIV/AIDS now than they were at the beginning of the crisis.
- It is important for teens to understand the link between HIV and sex and to know how to tell between myths and facts about HIV transmission.

Words to Understand

To be *closeted*, or in the closet, is when a gay person has not told his friends and family about his sexual orientation.

Grassroots organizations are created and supported by ordinary citizens, not governmental organizations.

MSM are men who have sex with men, which may or may not mean that they are gay. Some MSM identify as straight because their primary physical and emotional relationships are with women.

Sub-Saharan Africa is the part of the world most affected by AIDS. It includes all of the countries south of the Sahara desert, more than 50% of the continent of Africa.

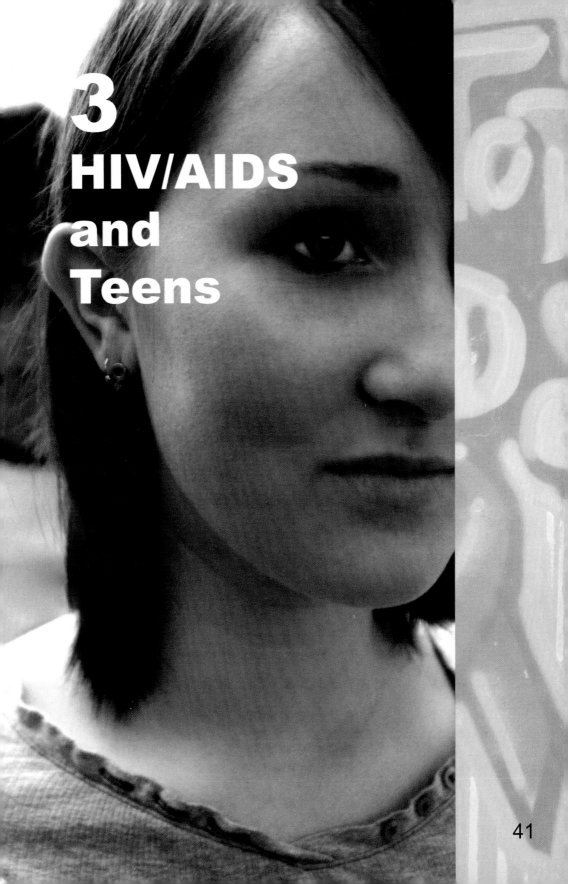

3
HIV/AIDS
and
Teens

41

There are approximately 33.2 million people living with HIV/AIDS in the world. That is four times the population of New York City, or sixteen times the population of Paris. Over two million of those people are children under the age of 15, and still more are young adults between the ages of 15 and 25. There are enough children with HIV/AIDS to populate a city and the numbers are still growing every year. Many teens think that HIV will not affect them, but every person needs to know that HIV does not discriminate because of age, sexuality, gender, or race. Teenagers can contract HIV by having unprotected sex or shooting up illegal drugs—even on their first time. Sometimes young people feel invincible because they are young and healthy, but that false sense of security won't protect them from the risks associated with heroin and other illicit drugs or adults who take advantage of teen boys or girls.

So what does HIV mean to you? It might already be in your life: affecting one of your friends, an uncle, or even

Anyone, no matter color, creed, sex, or orientation, can get HIV and AIDS; the disease does not discriminate.

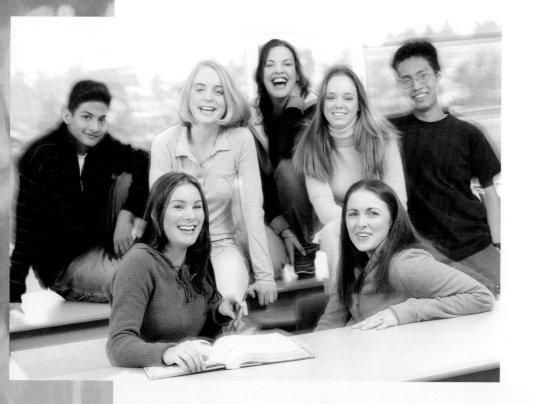

one of your parents. You may have heard about it in school or heard your friends talking, or even joking about it. Or, maybe you've heard about HIV/AIDS and know what it means, but don't know where it came from or how it might affect you someday.

A lot of teenagers don't understand how HIV is transmitted, so they will do things like joke about their friends having HIV, being gay, or being dirty. But being gay does not mean that a person has HIV, and having HIV does not mean a person is dirty. Some children were born with HIV because their mothers were infected with the virus, and some children, especially in developing countries, contract HIV at a young age through tainted transfusions or dirty needles used in medical procedures. Put yourself in the shoes of a person with HIV. How would you want to be treated? Does that change what you think of people with HIV/AIDS?

Early AIDS Crisis and Response

When HIV/AIDS was first discovered in the United States in the early 1980s, no one knew what was causing it or how it was spread. It was first called GRID, or Gay Related Immune Deficiency, because gay men were dying of mysterious cancers, pneumonia, and infections. It took a while for doctors to figure out that the disease was not just in the gay male population. Widespread HIV infection began in 1981, but the actual cause of the disease was not discovered until 1983, when two scientists, one in the United States and one in France, found the HIV virus at the same time. It wasn't until 1985 that a test was developed to screen the blood supply for HIV, so hemophiliacs and other people who received blood transfusions were often at risk for contracting HIV.

In the United States between the years of 1981 and 1985, no one knew that they had HIV until they started developing symptoms of AIDS. They didn't know why it seemed to target the gay population, or how to protect themselves from infection. Many organizations dedicated to helping the HIV-affected community sprung up, including ACT UP, Gay Men's Health Crisis (or GMHC), and numerous other **grassroots** programs designed to support and educate both AIDS patients and their communities. At the beginning of the AIDS crisis, young people, especially in the gay community, worked to make safer sex and education a top priority in preventing HIV/AIDS, and to provide support and understanding to AIDS patients.

HIV in the New Millennium

In the years since the beginning of the AIDS crisis, scientists have developed more and more effective drugs to make living with HIV manageable. There is a danger, though, that because of the new drugs some people might think they don't have to protect themselves from HIV anymore. Young people are less cautious about safer sex and sharing needles now than they were after HIV started spreading in the 1980s. Some teenagers believe that they are immune from HIV because it was only a problem in the 80s, or because they believe that there will be a vaccine soon enough that they don't have to worry about getting infected. Scientists have been trying to find a cure for AIDS since the beginning of the epidemic, but because HIV mutates so rapidly, it has been very difficult to even begin to develop a vaccine.

The role of teens in the AIDS epidemic is very important. Some people diagnosed in the early 1980s have lived with the disease for over twenty years, and still remember the terror that it caused when no one knew how or why it was spreading so quickly. But for the second generation of teenagers in a world with AIDS, HIV is not necessarily a death sentence. Because there are drugs like protease inhibitors and AZT that can keep HIV patients alive for decades, some young people believe that it's not important to guard against the infection. Some teens believe that it's not possible to get HIV if it's their first time having sex; others believe that it is better to get HIV because then they won't have to worry about preventing it anymore.

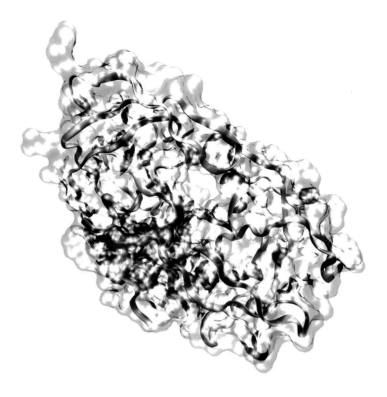

Because teens are one of the highest risk populations, it is important that they have access to information, condoms and other safer sex materials, and supportive parents, teachers, or friends who are willing to talk about their concerns and questions. There are also many online resources for teens that might not be comfortable talking with their parents about sex or drug use.

How HIV Can Affect Teens

In the United States, the population most affected by HIV is the gay community; however, in **Sub-Saharan Africa**, where the number of people affected by HIV/AIDS is over 22 million, more than 50% of HIV/AIDS patients are heterosexual women. Although many HIV/AIDS patients are adults, many people are likely to be infected when they are young. That is part of why HIV/AIDS is such a devastating disease: because it targets healthy young people, sapping their energy and leaving them susceptible

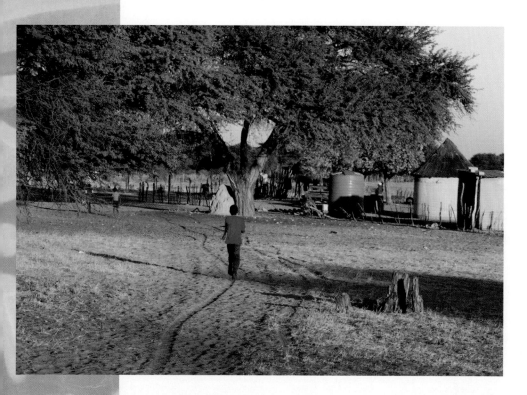

In Sub-Saharan Africa, whole villages have been devastated by the AIDS epidemic. Much of the time, this is because people are not educated about how to prevent the spread of this disease.

to serious infections and cancers. Even though some teens think that it might be better to just get HIV so they can stop worrying about it, they might not understand the realities of having HIV/AIDS. HIV patients must take a whole host of pills, deal with painful side effects, get their CD4 cells checked all the time, visit their doctors often, and deal with the emotional consequences of having a chronic disease that may take their lives someday. HIV-positive people can have busy and happy lives, but they must deal with their disease as well as people's reactions to the disease every step of the way. So while dealing with HIV is possible, it is still not something that anyone would willingly choose for themselves.

Gay Teens

It can be hard for gay teens to gain acceptance in any culture. It's difficult for any teen to handle the realities of being sexually active in today's world, and for gay teens it can be even more difficult to make the decision to come out. For some people, being gay is against their religious practices or cultural background, and they must endure homophobia, racism, or bigotry because of their sexuality. But because of the higher risk of HIV transmission in unprotected anal sex, it is important that men who have sex with men (*MSM*), whether they identify as gay, straight, or bisexual, are honest about their sexual activity and HIV status. If someone is **closeted**, it is much harder for him to be honest with his spouse or sexual partners, because he not only has to talk about his sexual history, but he also has to admit his sexual preference. In some countries, it is more acceptable to be gay than in others, but there are still acts of violence perpetrated against gay communities around the world because their societies don't understand or approve of them. For gay teens, it is especially important to learn about communication and respect in sexual relationships, because they are more at risk for transmitting HIV; it is also important for them to know the facts about HIV/AIDS because they are more likely to personally know someone who has the disease. Even though HIV/AIDS is not as scary as it was in the early 1980s, it is still a serious issue. The best way to help keep the youngest generation of gay teens safe from HIV/AIDS is to educate them, and to remain open and honest about what it means to be gay in a world with AIDS.

Heterosexual Teens

Although gay teens are more at risk for HIV because anal sex is a higher-risk activity than vaginal sex, heterosexual teens also need to understand the risks of having unprotected intercourse, which can transmit HIV as well as cause pregnancy. Straight or bisexual, sexually active teens need to be aware of birth control or other kinds of contraception as well as condoms, and they need to know that using one does not mean that it's not a good idea to use the other. Girls on birth control often think that it protects them from all of the risks of unprotected sex, not

Did You Know?

In a survey of almost 6,000 American MSM, 55% of men ages 15-22 did not tell anyone that they were sexually attracted to men. According to the CDC, which sponsored the survey, "MSM who do not disclose their sexual orientation are less likely to seek HIV testing, so if they become infected, they are less likely to know it."

just pregnancy. The truth is that it only affects hormones; it does not provide any type of barrier against HIV or other STIs. And although condoms are very effective at preventing HIV transmission, because of the chance of condom failure, it is always a good idea to use two types of contraception. That way, if a condom breaks, both partners will only have to worry about disease transmission, and not disease transmission with the possibility of pregnancy. If a girl does get pregnant, she should get tested for HIV as soon as possible, to protect her baby from infection. Straight partners should also know about the availability of emergency contraception in their area, so that they can deal with a broken condom without secondary contraception. Remember that neither birth control nor emergency contraception protects against HIV!

The pill, although it does prevent pregnancy and regulate periods, does not protect you from HIV.

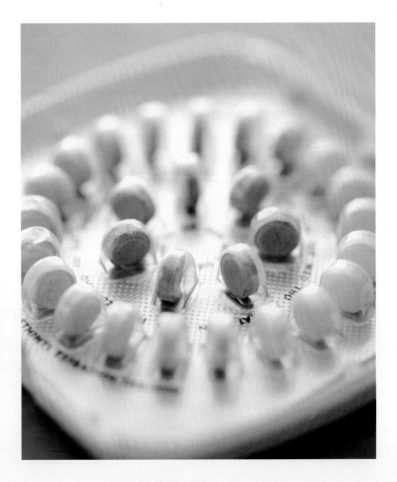

Real People

Alee Stirling was five years old when she became suddenly and unexplainably sick. After hospital visits and dozens of tests, the doctors still didn't know what was wrong with her. Shortly after her baby brother was born, he also became sick. The doctors decided to test both children and their mother for HIV. All three came back positive. Alee's mother Suzan had been living with HIV for almost a decade without knowing it: a previous boyfriend of hers had died of what he said was cancer, but was likely an AIDS-related infection. To protect her children, Suzan and her husband Clay decided to keep the family's HIV status a secret. Finally, in 2008, seventeen-year-old Alee decided that she wanted to share their story with the world. She and her brothers appeared on the cover of Poz, a magazine for HIV-positive people. Both Alee and her brother Mitchell have remained healthy, and in 2006, Suzan and Clay adopted an HIV-positive Ethiopian orphan named Yonas. The family's openness about their HIV status has made a statement about how you can be happy, healthy, and HIV-positive in a world that often doesn't understand what it means to have HIV.

In many countries, if a pregnant teen decides that she is not ready to have a baby she has the option of either having an abortion or putting the child up for adoption. If she is HIV-positive and decides to give up the child, she should still get proper prenatal care and take antiretroviral treatment to ensure that the baby is healthy.

Questions

Teens are likely to have a lot of questions about sex and the transmission of HIV. Misinformation from friends and a lack of understanding of the virus can lead to some misconceptions that keep teens from protecting themselves as well as they could. Here are some common questions that teens might have about HIV and sex.

I use condoms most of the time, except when I forget or I don't have them. Isn't using condoms sometimes better than never?

Yes, it is—but your risk of getting HIV goes up every time you have unprotected sex. By having protected sex sometimes, you are reducing the risk of giving or getting HIV from that partner, but you are still exposing yourself by having sex without condoms.

My boyfriend and I were both tested for HIV and it came out negative! Doesn't that mean that it's okay for my boyfriend to stop wearing a condom when we have sex?

No. It's great that you got yourself tested, but there a few reasons why you should still use protection.
First: when young people first start having relationships, it's very new and exciting! Everyone makes mistakes, though—and it's possible that your boyfriend won't always be faithful to you. If he isn't, and he doesn't use a condom, he could pass on HIV or other STIs to you.
Second: If you are not using birth control, then you should definitely keep using condoms to prevent pregnancy. If you are on the Pill, there is still a small risk of pregnancy, especially if you don't take it on time every day, or accidentally forget to take one. Consider whether you would be financially and emotionally ready to take care of a baby. If the answer is no, it's just another good reason to keep on using condoms.
Third: Again, it's great that you got yourself tested. But a negative test should never be a reason to celebrate or feel invincible—if you are engaging in unsafe sex or using injection drugs, there is still a much higher chance that you will contract HIV than if you are being careful.

One of my friends and I had unprotected sex. He told me afterwards that he has AIDS. But we didn't have anal sex and he didn't come in me, so I couldn't have gotten it, right?

No. Any unprotected sex, not just anal sex, can transmit HIV. Even though he didn't come in you, males produce fluid before ejaculating, often called pre-cum, that can contain both sperm and viral material. So even if he didn't ejaculate inside of you, it's still possible that you contracted HIV. You should go and get tested now, and get tested again when it has been three months, and again at six months. If it is negative all three times, then you didn't get HIV from him. And in the future, insist on a condom!

One of my friends told me that it's not possible to get HIV or STIs if you have unprotected sex during your period. Is this true?

No. Transmission of HIV or other STIs is actually more likely during your period, because the blood in menstrual fluid is a more powerful route of transmission than regular vaginal fluid. Your friend may have thought this because it is less likely for a woman to get pregnant during her period if she has unprotected sex—however, this is not always true, so it is an unreliable birth control method for teens.

A lot of girls at my school give boys oral sex instead of having regular sex. Are they safe from getting HIV?

Not necessarily; the risk is low compared to other types of sex, but there is still a small risk of infection. Transmission is more likely if the partner giving oral sex has any cuts or infections in his or her mouth. The person receiving oral sex is at very low risk unless the giver is actively bleeding from his mouth, since saliva does not have enough of the virus in it to transmit HIV. Although oral sex is not thought of as very high-risk sex, it is still important to protect yourself. There are flavored condoms available in many places, and they can be a pleasant way to protect yourself during oral sex.

STRAIGHT FROM THE SOURCE

(From "The UNGASS, Gender and Women's Vulnerability to HIV/AIDS in Latin America and the Caribbean," 2002 WHO document.)

Age mixing—older men having sex with young women— is another manifestation of unequal gender relations, especially prevalent in the Caribbean. Age-mixing is guided by two central factors: (1) the belief among men that younger women are more passive, more fertile, and less likely to be infected with HIV, and (2) the belief among young women that an older man will be a better and more stable economic provider for herself and her children. Though the practice of age-mixing pre-dates HIV/AIDS, it has significant consequences for the spread of the pandemic, placing young women at an increased risk of infection. In one Jamaican surveillance center for pregnant women, young women in their late teens had almost twice the HIV/AIDS prevalence rate of older women. Although most men are initially infected before the age of 25, older men have generally been sexually active longer and are therefore more likely to be already infected than younger males.

It has been well documented that men are less likely to seek health care than women, since they are socialized to believe that men do not get sick. This remains true for men who are infected with HIV/AIDS, even though the virus is easier to detect in men than in women. Men who do not use health services regularly, yet continue to engage in high-risk behaviour such as unprotected sex with multiple partners, place themselves and all of their partners at risk. Although in Latin America, there are more health services directed toward young men than in any other region, HIV/AIDS and STI services still tend to be offered within a broader reproductive health context, which targets women rather than men for health interventions, missing the needs of this most important population.

What Do You Think?

- According to this WHO document, why is age-mixing desirable to both young women and older men? What are the risks?

- Which group of people should health services target in order to reduce the transmission of HIV/AIDS in the Caribbean and Latin American countries?

- From what you've learned about the transmission of HIV/AIDS, do you think that the heterosexual women in this situation are more or less likely to contract HIV/AIDS from their sexual encounters than their male partners? Why?

Find Out More

HIV/AIDS can be a difficult subject for any teen to talk about with her friends or parents. If you don't feel comfortable talking to someone in your life, you should consider talking to someone at a family planning or HIV clinic. Remember that they are there to help and answer questions about HIV/AIDS, never to make you feel guilty or stupid about sex or HIV! Here are some online resources that may also be helpful in answering your questions.

www.avert.org/young.htm

www.thebody.com/index/whatis/children.html

aids.about.com/od/childrenteens/tp/teensandhiv.htm

www.cdc.gov/hiv/resources/Factsheets/youth.htm

Words to Understand

An *anaphylactic reaction* is when the body has a severe allergic reaction to a food, material, or insect bite or sting. The symptoms of anaphylaxis are difficulty breathing, swelling in the mouth or throat, dizziness, vomiting, and hives.

An *autoclave* is a machine that sterilizes equipment at high pressure and temperature. It works best on metal instruments, as plastics melt at high temperatures.

A *caesarean section* is a surgical procedure in which a baby is removed through making an incision in the mother's belly.

When a man is *circumcised*, the foreskin of his penis has been removed in a surgical procedure.

Ejaculate is the mixture of sperm and other sexual fluid that come out of a man when he orgasms.

If a material is *non-permeable*, it means that liquid cannot pass through it.

Serostatus is the presence or absense of antibodies in someone's blood.

Sharps include hypodermic needles, scalpels, and any other sharp objects usually used in the medical profession.

Spermicide is a chemical, usually in cream form, that kills sperm cells when applied before sexual intercourse.

A *viral load* is a measure of the number of copies of a virus in a given amount of blood, usually cubic millimeters.

Here's what you need to know

- Using safer sex practices is the best way to protect yourself from HIV.
- There are several different types of condoms, but only two are effective against HIV transmission.
- IV drug users should not share equipment, in order to protect themselves from HIV.
- Other types of drugs can lower inhibitions and lead to risky behaviors.
- Tattoos and piercings should be done in a sterile environment.
- Health care professionals have a special set of procedures to protect themselves from HIV.

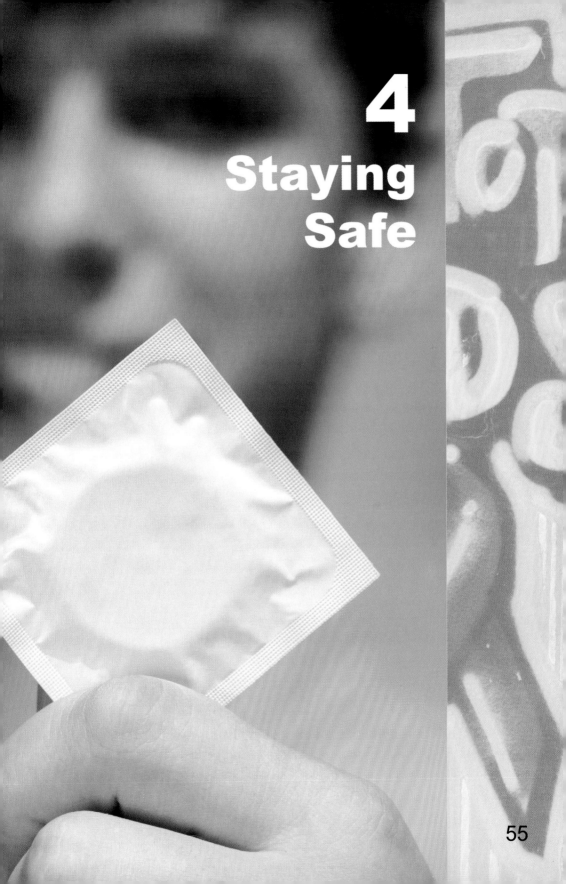

4
Staying
Safe

Now that you know how HIV is transmitted, you can learn about how to protect yourself from HIV exposure. Here are some of the things you can do to stay safe.

Safer Sex

Using safer sex practices is the easiest and most important way that you can protect yourself from HIV. Although the only completely safe sex is abstinence, there are a number of things you can do to limit your exposure if you choose to have sex. In any sexual contact, the best way to minimize risk is to know your sex partner, use condoms, and refrain from using drugs or alcohol during sex.

Condoms

For both heterosexual and homosexual couples, the most important barrier against HIV is the consistent use of condoms and lubrication. Condoms not only prevent pregnancy and the spreading of sexually transmitted infections, they can significantly reduce the chance of HIV infection, even between an HIV-positive and a healthy partner. There are two types of condoms: male and female. Male condoms, long sheaths of *non-permeable* material designed to fit over the penis and prevent *ejaculate* from entering the receiving partner's body, are the more commonly used of the two. The female condom is a similar sheath that is designed to fit in the receiving partner's vagina or anus, although it is less reliable for anal intercourse than a male condom; it can be a good alternative to the male condom for partners who are unwilling or unable to wear male condoms. Male and female condoms should not be worn at the same time, as they can get caught on each other during sex. Some people think that using more than one male condom at a time will provide extra protection against both pregnancy and STI's, but this is not true. Never wear more than one male condom at a time: two condoms will rub against each other and break easily. Condoms will sometimes break during sex even if used correctly. If this happens, remove the broken condom and put on a new one as soon as possible. Do not stop using condoms just because one broke! Condoms are much more effective at preventing disease transmission than unprotected sex, even if they fail sometimes. Condom failure does not guarantee transmission. Replace the condom before continuing to have sex.

Latex

The most common and effective type of condom is the latex condom. If used correctly, the condom will prevent both sperm and viral agents from passing through the

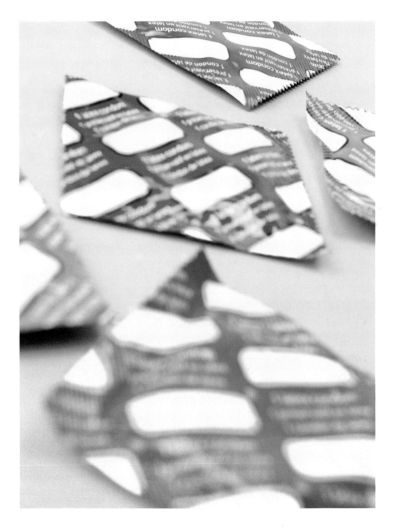

There are many different kinds of condoms, including ones made out of polyurethane for people who are allergic to latex.

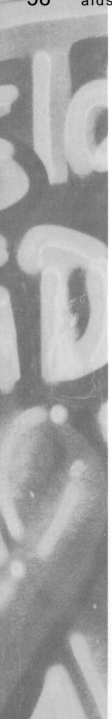

condom during sex. They are relatively inexpensive and available in many places. Family planning agencies and universities or colleges often provide latex condoms to clients or students for no charge. Do not use latex condoms that have been in direct sunlight, under physical stress, or that have been opened. Oil-based lubricants break down latex and should not be used with latex condoms.

Polyurethane

Some people are allergic to latex, which can cause symptoms ranging from itchiness to a life-threatening *anaphylactic reaction*. In this case, polyurethane condoms are recommended. The reason that polyurethane condoms are not recommended for people without latex allergies is because they tend to be looser and to slip off the penis more easily, which increases the risk of disease transmission; however, if both partners are aware of this, the polyurethane condom can be used with the same degree of effectiveness as a latex. Polyurethane condoms can be used with oil or water-based lubricants.

Natural Membrane

Natural membrane or lambskin condoms are made out of the intestines of sheep. Although they are effective at preventing pregnancy, they do not protect against sexually transmitted infections, including HIV.

Lubrication

Using lubricant is an important but often overlooked part of safer sex practices. Condoms often break during sex because of too much friction, when the movement of the penis against the vagina or anus creates so much heat that the condom is weakened to the point of breaking. Lubrication draws the heat away and keeps the condom intact. It also prevents vaginal or anal tearing that might result from un-lubricated sex and provide a pathway for virus transmission. Avoid lubricant or spermicide that contains

Nonoxynol-9, as it can irritate the skin and create lesions that lead to higher risk of transmission of HIV.

Circumcision

Studies have shown that female-to-male transmission is reduced by almost 50% when the male is *circumcised*. There are several reasons an uncircumcised man has a higher risk of getting HIV from a woman: the foreskin is easily torn because it is a flap of skin, allowing a route to the bloodstream for the virus; it is a mucous membrane, which provides a moist environment for HIV to reproduce; and there tends to be a higher rate of STIs in uncircumcised men, which can also lead to an increased rate of HIV transmission. Circumcision may be a good preventative measure in developing countries or where condoms may not be available. However, if condoms are an option, using them is a far more effective preventative measure than circumcision.

Women and Confidence

In many societies, men are still considered more important than women, which can complicate heterosexual relations when it comes to preventing HIV. A woman might not have the power to demand that her partner wear condoms, or to ask about his *serostatus*, which can increase her risk of infection. In any society, it is important for a woman to feel confident enough to ask questions that can protect her health. It can be helpful to talk to a counselor or trusted friend, whether it is at a school, a hospital or clinic, or at home. Although many programs teach abstinence education rather than educating their students about condoms and safer sex, it is important for both men and women to know that sex is a natural part of life—but also that there are risks, and it is a good idea to understand and know how to minimize those risks. Not being educated about sex may increase abstinence, but it can also decrease knowledge for people who want to be sexually active. It is especially important for women to know how to protect themselves, so that they can share that knowledge with a male partner who might refuse to wear condoms because "they don't feel as good."

Protection from Drug-Related Exposure

Using dirty needles to inject drugs is one of the most common ways that people get HIV. But heroin and other injection drugs are not the only drugs that lead to HIV exposure–alcohol, marijuana, and other recreational drugs contribute to risky sexual behavior and poor judgment, which can lead to infection through unsafe sex. The best way to stay healthy is to abstain from drugs altogether, but if you decide to use them, there are some things that you can do to minimize your risk.

Staying Safe During Intravenous Injection

Never share equipment with anyone else, not even a close friend. Equipment includes cotton, water, needles, and

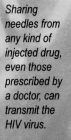

Sharing needles from any kind of injected drug, even those prescribed by a doctor, can transmit the HIV virus.

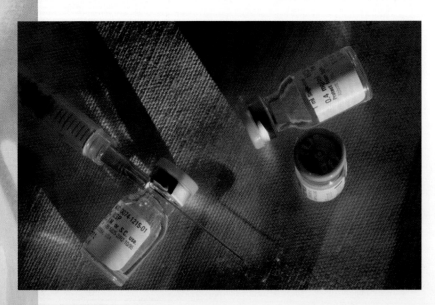

other drug paraphernalia—anything that touches blood or touches something else that had contact with blood should never be shared. Heroin users are not the only people at risk, either: injecting steroids, cocaine, speed, or any other type of drug carries a risk of transmitting both HIV and Hepatitis C. If you do inject drugs, do not share needles. If you must share needles, rinse them with water, clean them with bleach three times, and rinse them again with clean water. The best way to keep from contracting HIV through injection drugs is to stop. Rehabilitation programs can help wean you off of the drugs and let you live a healthy, drug-free life.

Staying Safe While Using Other Drugs

Alcohol, marijuana, and cocaine are some drugs that people commonly use in social settings. In many countries, there is an age limit on alcohol use, and marijuana and cocaine are illegal in most countries. Using any one of these drugs, or other recreational drugs like ecstasy or methamphetamines, reduces your awareness and lowers your inhibitions. Some of them can even cause you to black out and forget entire periods of time, including sexual experiences. In order to protect yourself while using any of these drugs, it is a good idea to be with people you know and trust, or to ask a sober friend to keep an eye on you.

Tattoos and Body Piercings

Although people often worry about the risk of transmission through tattoos and body piercings, the likelihood of contracting HIV in either of these ways is very low. Most tattoo parlors have procedures to sterilize their equipment and prevent infection. If you are interested in getting a tattoo or piercing and have concerns about the risks, feel free to ask questions at the tattoo parlor. Most piercers and tattoo artists have extensive training, wear latex gloves during any procedure, use special machines called *auto-claves* to sterilize their equipment, throw away needles

Did You Know?

If a woman takes the appropriate antiretroviral treatment during pregnancy, her risk of transmitting HIV to her child is less than 2%. Without HIV treatment, mother-to-child transmission is about 25% likely.

after one use, and are inspected by health departments routinely in order to ensure safety.

Do not try to tattoo or pierce yourself at home, whether by yourself or by a friend! Any piercing or tattooing implements used in the home will not be sterile, which can not only transmit Hepatitis C or HIV, but also bacteria that can cause painful or even life-threatening infections.

Preventing Mother-to-Child Exposure

The first step in preventing transmission from a mother to her baby is to test the mother when she first becomes pregnant, or before she becomes pregnant if possible. If the mother is HIV-positive, she can be given a course of anti-retroviral medication during her pregnancy and labor that will keep her *viral load* low and prevent transmission to her baby. If she is properly medicated during her pregnancy, the mother can also give birth vaginally rather than through a *caesarean section* without risking exposure. Lastly, it is important that women in countries that have access to clean water and formula do not breastfeed, in order to keep their babies from contracting HIV through breast milk. In developing countries, a doctor can help make the mother make the decision whether to breastfeed or use formula, depending on the safety of the water supply. The baby will also be given anti-retroviral therapy after birth and checked for HIV every few months.

Preventing HIV Exposure in Medical Settings

Health-care employees must exercise universal precautions when treating all patients, not just ones with HIV. One of these precautions is the use of latex gloves when touching potentially infectious fluid (blood, semen, any bodily fluid that contains blood), mucous membranes, or material that has come into contact with infectious fluid. More precautions include the use of gowns, goggles, and needle-stick prevention guidelines as appropriate. Needles are never to be re-capped, reused, bent, broken, removed from their syringe, or otherwise handled to prevent needle-stick injuries. Goggles and gowns are used during procedures that are likely to splash blood or fluid onto the health care worker. All disposable *sharps* are thrown away in special sharps containers marked with biological hazard stickers.

Hygiene

In general, although the risk of spreading HIV from casual contact is very low, there is a risk of transmitting HIV if you share any items that may have contact with blood. Razors, tooth-brushes, and tweezers should not be shared. It is not only good hygiene to avoid using other people's personal products, but it can prevent other types of infections that could be passed through un-sterilized equipment.

Other

Some people engage in a ritual where they become "blood brothers"—both people cut their skin and mix their blood to symbolize their friendship or loyalty. This is a very risky behavior, and should never be practiced, even if both people are HIV-negative. There are other blood-borne infections that could be passed on during the ritual, especially Hepatitis B and C.

HIV Testing

Another way that you can protect yourself and others is to get tested for HIV every so often, or after any possible exposure. Remember that HIV tests are most effective when it has been at least three months since the exposure; also

Ask the Doctor

Q: I'm a 19-year-old gay man. When I was in high school, I injected heroin and was infected with HIV. It's been two years since I was diagnosed and I have met another HIV-positive man who wants to be with me. We use condoms, but we've talked about having unprotected sex since we both have HIV. Would this be safe?

No. Even though you and your partner both have HIV, it's possible that you have two different mutations of the virus, or subtypes. There are two main types of HIV: HIV-1 and HIV-2. HIV-2 is only common in West Africa, but HIV-1 is the main type in the rest of the world. Even within HIV-1, there are many subtypes of the virus. It changes rapidly, sometimes creating two or more different strains within a single person. If you and your partner were to have unprotected sex, it is possible that your already weakened immune system would allow you to contract another, slightly different form of HIV. This is called superinfection, or coinfection, and it can make HIV progress to AIDS faster than usual. It's great that you are already using condoms—and the best way for you to stay healthy is to keep on doing just that.

remember that a negative HIV test is no longer valid if you have unprotected sex with someone new. If you use a condom every time you have sex, discuss your HIV status with your partner, and get tested routinely, you can keep both yourself and your partner safe from HIV. If you need to know where to go to get tested, talk to your doctor; or, if you are in the United States, go to www.harvest.org to find a testing location near you. Remember that getting tested doesn't mean you have HIV or that you are a bad person—it means that you are being responsible and respectful of your health!

Safety for HIV Positive People

Although there are a lot of things that HIV-negative people can do to prevent exposure to HIV, it is also important for HIV-positive people to know how to protect themselves and their loved ones. The first is to take their medication every day to help keep their illness from progressing. Another is to practice safer sex, even with another HIV-positive person. It is possible for two people with HIV to have several different strains in their body, and if they exchange bodily fluids, the different HIV infections can stack on top of each other and create an even stronger infection. Both HIV-positive and HIV-negative people have a responsibility to talk about their HIV status before engaging in sexual intercourse. Some people disagree, saying that HIV-positive people already have enough to deal with without having to admit to healthy people that they have HIV; others argue that HIV-negative people trust that an HIV-positive person would disclose their status before risking exposure.

Precautions After Possible HIV Exposure

Some medical systems have special medication that they can give you if you were exposed to HIV accidentally, through a sexual assault, an incident with a broken con-

Real People

In 1991, Magic Johnson was a successful basketball player who played for the LA Lakers. He had won numerous MVP awards, set records, and became a legend of basketball in his thirteen-year career. He was also known for his magnetic personality and constant cheerfulness. However, on November 8th, 1991 he announced his immediate retirement. He had learned the day before that he was infected with HIV. At that time, HIV was still seen as a disease of drug users and gay people, so when Johnson, a straight, famous basketball player, announced his HIV status, the world became more aware that HIV could affect anyone.

In the years since his diagnosis, Johnson has created his own foundation in order to support small non-profit organizations that provide scholarships to underprivileged youth as well as HIV/AIDS education to children and young adults.

dom and known HIV-positive partner, or needle-stick injury. It is important that if you think you were exposed to HIV that you receive this treatment within 72 hours after exposure. This treatment is called Post-Exposure Prophylaxis, or PEP.

STRAIGHT FROM THE SOURCE

(From "Adult Male Circumcision Significantly Reduces Risk of Acquiring HIV", NIH article, 2006)

The National Institute of Allergy and Infectious Diseases (NIAID), part of the National Institutes of Health (NIH), announced an early end to two clinical trials of adult male circumcision because an interim review of trial data revealed that medically performed circumcision significantly reduces a man's risk of acquiring HIV through heterosexual intercourse. The trial in Kisumu, Kenya, of 2,784 HIV-negative men showed a 53 percent reduction of HIV acquisition in circumcised men relative to uncircumcised men, while a trial of 4,996 HIV-negative men in Rakai, Uganda, showed that HIV acquisition was reduced by 48 percent in circumcised men. . . .

The findings from the African studies may have less impact on the epidemic in the United States for several reasons. In the United States, most men have been circumcised. Also, there is a lower prevalence of HIV. Moreover, most infections among men in the United States are in men who have sex with men, for whom the amount of benefit provided by circumcision is unknown. Nonetheless, the overall findings of the African studies are likely to be broadly relevant regardless of geographic location: a man at sexual risk who is uncircumcised is more likely than a man who is circumcised to become infected with HIV. Still, circumcision is only part of a broader HIV prevention strategy that includes limiting the number of sexual partners and using condoms during intercourse.

What Do You Think?

- According to this NIH document, how effective is circumcision in preventing HIV transmission during heterosexual intercourse?

- Why might circumcision be a more practical prevention tool in Africa than in the United States?

- Why do you think that the researchers stopped the clinical trail early?

Find Out More

To find out more about HIV prevention and precautions, check out these Web sites:

www.cdcnpin.org/scripts/hiv/prevent.asp

www.thebody.com/index/safesex.html

www.sfaf.org/aids101/hiv_disease.html

www.iwannaknow.org/basics2/hiv_aids.html

www.cdc.gov/ncidod/dhqp/bp_universal_precautions.html

Here's what you need to know

• HIV reproduces by injecting its genetic material inside a cell, making copies of itself, and leaving the cell again.

• There are five different kinds of drugs that target HIV by interfering with different stages of the copying process.

• HAART treatment consists of two or more HIV drugs used as a daily regimen to fight HIV/AIDS.

• Doctors assess CD4 counts, viral load, and the presence of opportunistic infections in order to decide on a treatment plan.

• It is important for HIV patients to take their treatment, to eat healthy, and to exercise.

• Some people don't believe that HIV/AIDS exists, which only hurts the world's efforts to prevent millions of deaths from HIV.

5
HIV
Treatment

When AIDS was first discovered, the only treatments for the disease were the treatments for the **opportunistic infections** like Pneumocystis Carinii Pneumonia and Kaposi's sarcoma. But as scientists started to understand more about what caused AIDS, and after an HIV test was created, they also started working on drugs that could help treat HIV and prevent AIDS from developing. Many of these drugs are very toxic, causing kidney and liver damage, and some people develop resistance to them. But medications prolong the lives of HIV/AIDS patients, making it possible for them to live with their disease for decades.

HIV Structure and Drugs

In order to understand how these drugs work, it is important to know how the HIV virus works. HIV is a retrovirus, which means that it has a special shape and function that is different than that of more typical viruses. HIV has two strands of **RNA** in its core, surrounded by protease and reverse transcriptase. It is encased by a viral envelope, which is covered in little spikes. Most viruses replicate using DNA, so the fact that HIV uses RNA to copy itself means that the copying process is a little more complicated. The RNA in HIV has only nine genes, as opposed to humans or even bacteria, which can have hundreds or thousands of genes.

The way HIV infects a CD4 cell is by bumping into it and sticking to it because of the little spikes on the viral envelope. After the virus and the cell have stuck together, the virus injects its contents into the cell, leaving the empty envelope behind. Inside the cell, HIV starts using its RNA and reverse transcriptase to convert RNA into **DNA**, which is compatible with the human cell. Once the HIV DNA is created, the cell integrates it into its own DNA. Once this has happened, any time the cell reproduces by copying messenger RNA out of its DNA, it also makes copies of the imposter HIV DNA. After the messenger RNA has been created, it can exit the cell and create more HIV-infected material. When the messenger

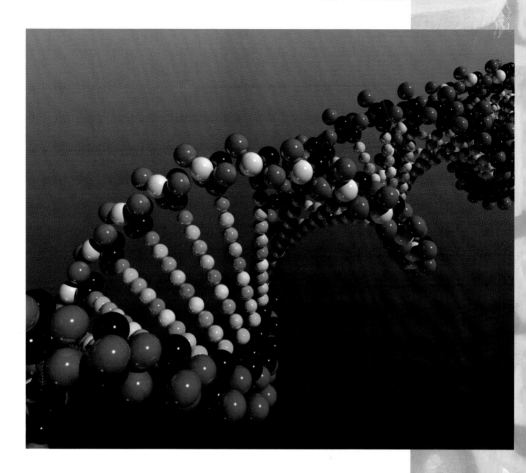

RNA was made, HIV genetic material is also produced within the RNA and chopped out into individual pieces by the protease molecules. Once all of these things have happened, the HIV-infected genetic material is ready to bud from the cell, mature, and infect more cells.

All HIV drugs work by interfering with different stages of the copying process. They cannot eliminate HIV, but they can keep it from infecting more and more cells.

Medications

There are five basic types of HIV drugs that people can take to help keep their HIV infections under control. The first, AZT, came out in the late 1980s, and new medications are still being developed.

Many viruses consist of DNA, like every other organism. HIV, however, consists only of two strands of RNA. This means that HIV has only nine genes, unlike other organisms, which have thousands of different genes.

Nucleoside/Nucleotide Reverse Transcriptase Inhibitors, or NRTIs

The HIV virus, a retrovirus, reproduces using a special enzyme called the reverse transcriptase enzyme. NRTIs interfere with the reverse transcriptase DNA reproduction process so that the virus finishes copying its DNA, but creates a mistake in the DNA so that it can't function. AZT, the first HIV drug available on the market, is an NRTI. They are still the most commonly used type of antiretroviral drug, and often at least two types of NRTIs are used in a typical HIV treatment program. NRTIs are often called "nukes," short for nucleoside or nucleotide.

Non-Nucleoside/Nucleotide Reverse Transcriptase Inhibitors, or NNRTIs

NNRTIs work in a similar way to NRTIs, by interfering with reverse transcriptase to stop HIV reproduction. However, NNRTIs work by preventing reverse transcriptase from functioning properly, so it can't even begin to copy the HIV RNA. NNRTIs are often called "non-nukes."

Protease Inhibitors

AZT and other NRTIs were first introduced in the late 1980s, but protease inhibitors were not discovered until the late 1990s. Protease acts like a pair of scissors, cutting the viral proteins into individual pieces. Protease inhibitors interfere with protease and keep it from cutting the long proteins into smaller HIV proteins.

Fusion or Entry Inhibitors

Fusion inhibitors keep HIV from getting inside immune cells, so it never even begins the copying process. It does this by interfering with the surface of the immune cell, making it so that the virus can't attach. These drugs cannot be taken in pill form because they would be digested in the stomach, so they are injected.

Integrase Inhibitors

This drug also interferes with the function of HIV, making it so that the HIV can't inject itself into the cell. If HIV can't insert its genetic material into the cell, then it can't infect new cells. This class of drugs is relatively new, released in the United States in late 2007 and in the United Kingdom in early 2008.

Combination Drugs

There are some pills that combine fixed doses of two different HIV medications that have already been proven to help HIV patients remain healthy. Fixed-dose combination pills can be helpful to people who want to take fewer pills, and because HIV patients often have to take many pills on a strict schedule, a combination drug can be very helpful in simplifying their routine. Combination drugs are not recommended for people under the age of 18, since the dose cannot be changed and children and teens usually need less medication than adults.

HAART

When three or more of these drugs are combined in a regimen for patients with HIV, it is called Highly Active Antiretroviral Therapy, or HAART. NRTIs are used as the basis of this treatment—usually, two different types of NRTIs are used in a standard HAART. The other drugs in HAART might include an NNRTI or a protease inhibitor. As in treatment for any disease, it is up to the patient to decide when to begin treatment. HAART can cause organ damage or result in drug resistant HIV in the patient, so it is important that the patient understand the benefits and risks of HAART. Remember that HAART is a treatment to prevent HIV from advancing to AIDS;

Did You Know?

Some people don't get sick even when their CD4 count is low, but it's much more likely that they will get an opportunistic infection. Other people have frequent complications even when their CD4 count is high.

it is not a cure, and can have long-term side effects even when used correctly.

When Should I Begin Treatment?

There are a few different things that doctors look for when they are considering HAART for their patients. There are three common tests that help doctors assess whether it is a good idea to start treatment.

CD4 Count

CD4 lymphocytes, also called T-cells, are the immune system's helper cells that fight infections and other stresses. They are also the cells that HIV infects. A normal person has thousands of CD4 cells in every cubic millimeter of blood, but people with HIV/AIDS often have only hundreds, leaving them open to infections that their bodies can't fight off.

Viral Load

Doctors also measure the viral load in an HIV infected person's blood to tell if the disease is progressing. Viral

This picture shows how the HIV virus uses T cells to reproduce in the human body. The virus invades the T cells, meaning that they are unable to fight off other, potentially dangerous infections.

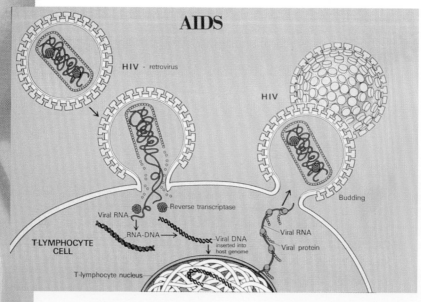

load is a term for the number of copies of HIV that are present in a cubic millimeter of blood. People with HIV can have less than a hundred up to millions of copies of the virus in a drop of their blood. If their viral load is low enough, it is called undetectable, meaning that they have fewer copies of the virus in their blood than is necessary for the test to be able to measure. It does not mean that there is no longer HIV in their blood, but it is a good thing.

Opportunistic Infections

Also referred to as OIs, opportunistic infections are infections or cancers that are rare in healthy people, but relatively common in HIV/AIDS patients. Patients with HIV are often not diagnosed with AIDS until they are diagnosed with an opportunistic infection, which is the reason that certain infections are also called **AIDS-defining conditions**. There are over twenty opportunistic infections that AIDS patients can get, but here are a few infections and other diseases that are very common in AIDS patients.

- Fungal infections, including thrush, also known as candidiasis, and cryptococcosis. Thrush is a fungal infection that presents as white patches in the mouth, although it can also infect the throat and intestinal tract. It often makes it very painful for the patient to eat. Cryptococcosis is a fungus that infects the brain, leading to meningitis, which can be fatal.
- Kaposi's sarcoma, a previously rare type of cancer that presents as blue or purple lesions on the skin.
- Tuberculosis, a disease affecting the lungs. It is infectious and very dangerous.
- Viral infections, such as the different kinds of herpes viruses, which can cause painful lesions on any part of the body. Hepatitis is another virus that can occur as a co-infection with HIV, especially in IV drug users.

- Pneumocystis Carinii Pneumonia, or PCP, is the most common and life-threatening infection in AIDS patients.
- Protozoa infections such as toxoplasmosis, which infects the brain.

All opportunistic infections can be very serious for HIV/AIDS patients. Technically, people who die from AIDS actually die from opportunistic infections that were able to get into their system because AIDS weakened their immune response. Some of these infections are only contagious to *immunosuppressed* patients such as the very old and very young but some of them are contagious to everyone, like hepatitis and herpes.

What does this mean for treatment? It means that if a patient with HIV presents with one of these infections or diseases, he should seriously consider starting on HAART.

If you think you have HIV, you should get tested immediately. It might be scary to think about having HIV, but if you found out early enough, you are much more likely to be able to treat your HIV and keep it from developing into AIDS for a long time.

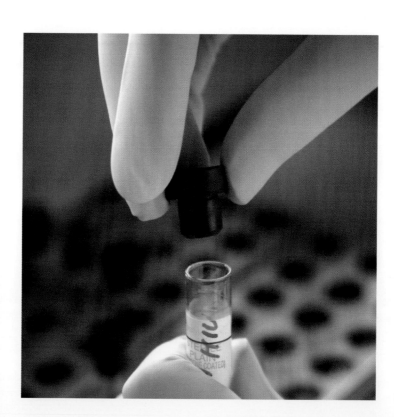

Deciding On Treatment

All treatments for HIV/AIDS require time and dedication. Many treatments have painful side effects, but can help keep HIV under control. Patients should discuss different combinations of drugs with their doctors, and weigh the good and bad effects of different treatments. Most treatments require that the patient take pills at a certain time every day, or that they take many pills throughout the day, both of which can be difficult for some people. Once a patient has begun HIV treatment, it is likely that he will be continuing it for the rest of his life. Children may also need to be on an HIV medication regimen, especially children who were born with the virus. Their immune systems are not as strong as an adult's, so it may be necessary to start treatment earlier.

Treatment Cost

Although HIV treatment can prolong the lives of HIV/AIDS patients for years or even decades, there are serious issues of cost—both economic and physical. In developed countries, the yearly cost of HIV treatment can be over $10,000. The cost varies in developing countries. Developed countries sometimes argue that *pharmaceutical companies* should lower the price of HIV drugs in order to save more lives in developing countries, but this topic can be *controversial*.

Side Effects

Some side effects of HIV treatment are unpleasant but manageable, and some side effects can be more serious. Doctors stress how important it is not to miss doses of any medications because the body can become allergic to HIV medication very quickly, and missing even one dose can result in the development of an allergy. If the patient takes the medication again, he might have an allergic reaction that can be painful or even fatal.

Real People

Charles Sako was training to become a primary school teacher in Kenya when he started getting sick all the time. He was afraid of getting kicked out of school, so he kept on putting off an HIV test. Finally, one of his doctors was worried enough that he tested Charles. The test came back positive.

Charles was devastated: what would happen to his brother and his mother, who had given up so much to send Charles to school? He left school and started living with a friend, but he soon got sicker. Then, one day, Charles met a counselor from Medecins Sans Frontieres (MSF), known as Doctors Without Borders in the United States, a program that provides health care and disaster relief in almost sixty countries around the world. The counselor got Charles on antiretroviral drugs, which helped Charles get healthier.

Today, Charles supports his family, volunteers with MSF, and has found companionship with a woman who is also HIV positive. Although people with HIV face many setbacks, Charles is an example of someone who has found happiness and purpose even after his diagnosis.

(From news.bbc.co.uk/2/shared/spl/hi/picture_gallery/05/africa_my_life_with_hiv/html/2.stml)

The mild side effects of HIV medication can include nausea, vomiting, diarrhea, tiredness, and headaches. Many HIV medications also change the appearance and location of fat on the body, leading to fat deposits on the body and thinning of the fat on the face. More serious side effects include anemia, liver damage, osteoporosis, and the onset of high cholesterol or diabetes. Patients must also tell their doctors what other medications they take, since HIV treatments can interfere with other drugs.

What Else Can I Do?

Because HIV patients get infections more easily than people with healthy immune systems, they should do as much as possible to eat healthy foods and get exercise. Patients with HIV should not eat foods that contain mold, or foods that might be spoiled, since it is more likely that they will develop fungal or bacterial infections from food sources. Adhering to medication regimens is also very important, since some of the medications only work if you take them at the same time every day, and if you never miss a dose.

AIDS Denialists

Some people believe that HIV does not lead to AIDS, HIV tests are inaccurate, or that HIV medications like AZT kill their patients. While it is true that HIV progresses to AIDS more slowly for some patients, usually because of HIV medications, millions of people have died from opportunistic infection brought on by HIV/AIDS; it is irresponsible and incorrect to claim that all of these people died from separate, non-HIV-related causes. HIV tests are over 99% accurate, and AZT, though it can be toxic, has helped to bring down the rate of mother-child transmission of HIV from 25% to less than 2% and extended the lives of hundreds of thousands of patients. It is unclear what conspiracy theorists intend to gain in denying the connections between HIV and AIDS. Misinformation from these sources is highly inflammatory, meant to draw controversy or to provide justification to people who are in denial of their HIV status. Remember that whatever the opinions of people who don't believe in HIV/AIDS may be, the realities of the HIV/AIDS crisis in Africa as well as the United States' devastating introduction to HIV/AIDS in the early 1980s is more than enough reason to practice safer sex and drug use.

STRAIGHT FROM THE SOURCE

(From unaids.org, "HIV Treatment")

HIV is an uncommon type of virus called a retrovirus, and drugs developed to disrupt the action of HIV are known as antiretrovirals or ARVs. These come in a variety of formulations designed to act on different stages of the life cycle of HIV.

The AIDS virus mutates rapidly, which makes it extremely skilful at developing resistance to drugs. To minimize this risk, people with HIV are generally treated with a combination of ARVs that attack the virus on several fronts at once.

The introduction of ARVs in 1996 transformed the treatment of HIV and AIDS, improving the quality and greatly prolonging the lives of many infected people in places where the drugs are available. Nevertheless, ARVs are not a cure. If treatment is discontinued the virus becomes active again, so a person on ARVs must take them for life.

Although the price of ARVs has fallen significantly in recent years, their cost remains an obstacle to access in the developing world. Moreover, the health infrastructure required to deliver antiretroviral therapy is lacking in many places. Of the estimated 6.5 million people in need of antiretroviral treatment, in June 2006, 1.65 million people were reported to have had access to ARV treatment in low- and middle-income countries (WHO, Jun2006).

Access to drugs depends not only on financial and human resources. It depends also on people who need them being aware of their HIV status, knowledgeable about treatment, and empowered to seek it.

Thus public information and education are important elements in widening access, alongside efforts to build or strengthen the health services.

The campaign for universal access to life saving drugs for HIV and AIDS, started originally by grassroots AIDS activists, is today a major focus of attention of UN agencies and others influential organizations at national and global levels.

What Do You Think?

- What are the greatest obstacles for developing countries in getting ARV treatment for their citizens?

- Why is it important to continue taking ARV treatment once you have begun?

- What is universal access and why is it important?

Find Out More

To find out more about HIV/AIDS treatments and symptoms, check out these Web sites:

www.aidsinfo.nih.gov/

www.thebody.com/content/art40477.html

A complete list of AIDS-defining conditions in Appendix B of this Web document: www.cdc.gov/MMWR/preview/MMWRhtml/00018871.htm

Here's what you need to know

- HIV might seem like a far-away problem, but it can actually affect any person at any time.
- If a family member, friend, or partner has HIV/AIDS, it's important that you support him and let him know that you love him.
- A loved one with HIV/AIDS might want to be private about her feelings about her illness.
- It is possible to have a sexual relationship with an HIV positive person, but you must always practice safer sex.
- You can help the cause of HIV/AIDS by contributing money or time to an HIV/AIDS organization or participating in AIDS education or World AIDS Day programs.

Words to Understand

Something that is *endemic* belongs to a certain region of the world. It often refers to diseases.

Something that is *epidemic* affects an unusually large number of a certain population. It also refers to diseases.

A *role model* is a person who provides inspiration through their accomplishments or actions, often to children and teens.

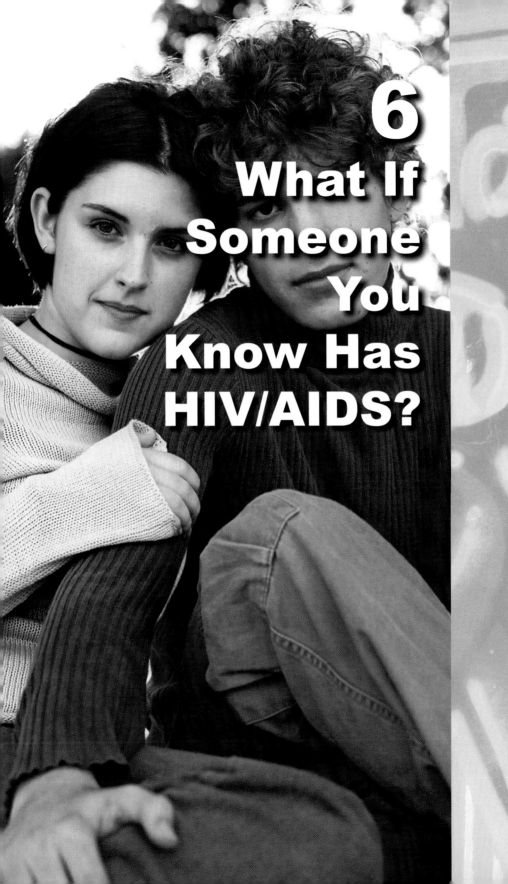

6
What If Someone You Know Has HIV/AIDS?

For some people, it might seem like HIV/AIDS is a distant problem. They might think that only people in big cities, people in Africa, or gay people get HIV. But the truth is that HIV can affect any person at any time and place. It is important to protect yourself, but it is also important to be educated, and to know that people with HIV/AIDS are very much the same as you, with ambitions, worries, passion, and wisdom.

Family

What if someone in your family has HIV/AIDS? It might be your brother, or your mom, or your uncle. It is important for you to know that HIV is not transmitted through casual contact: you can eat off of the same dishes or share food with an HIV-positive person; hug, kiss, or touch him; and share the same bathroom with him. People with HIV have to deal with a lot of things that HIV-negative people never even have to think about. They have to go to the doctor all the time, be careful about what they eat, and make many decisions based on the fact that they have HIV. On top of their health problems, they often have to deal with intolerance from people who don't understand HIV, as well as their own emotions of guilt, shame, or sadness. Remember that no one deserves HIV. No matter how your family member might have contracted the disease, it is not her fault. If someone you love has HIV or AIDS, it's very important to show that you love her, that you don't judge her for having HIV, and that you support her in both good times and bad. You might have to help out with her care—but be aware that every person deals with illness differently, and she may want to be private about how she is feeling.

Friends

As with any person you care about who has HIV, it is important to be supportive of a friend with HIV. This might include going with him to his doctor or hospital

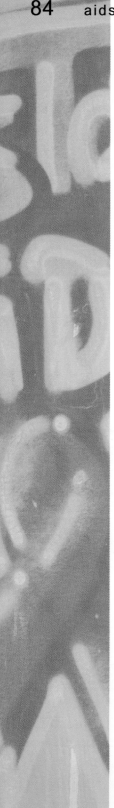

appointments, taking care of pets while he is away, or just being there to talk when your friend needs it. Hopefully, your friend has a family who can take care of him while he is sick, but sometimes families are not understanding about HIV, especially when their child is gay. If that's the case with one of your friends, he might call on you to be his family because his own family isn't there for him. Do what you can to help him, but also be mindful of your own needs because it's challenging for any person to take care of a sick person. If you find yourself overwhelmed, consider enlisting other friends for help, or find someone you trust that you can talk to about taking care of your friend.

Sexual Partners or Significant Others

If someone you are dating has HIV, it is more than possible to have a strong, loving relationship with her, both sexually and emotionally. You may have to take care of her sometimes, in the same way that you would take care of a sick friend or family member, but often it's more complicated to care for someone with whom you are intimate. An HIV-positive person might ask her partner to let her be independent about taking her own medications and other medical treatments, or she might ask her partner to help by setting an alarm to take medication or provide comfort when she is sick. It depends on whether she is comfortable sharing her feelings and concerns about HIV with her partner—it is natural for an HIV-positive person to desire privacy about her health, even with someone she cares about.

Whether you are HIV-negative or positive, both you and your HIV-positive partner need to practice safer sex at all times. Sometimes when two people are comfortable in a relationship, they don't use safer sex practices all the time, or may even stop using them altogether; however, it is especially important that any couple with at least one HIV-positive partner be very careful. It only takes one incident of unprotected sex to contract HIV, which both partners would have to deal with for the rest of their lives. People who don't have the same HIV status can face difficulties that are not common in relationships with two HIV-negative people, but these problems can be overcome if both partners are honest and respectful of each other. It is also possible for a couple with different HIV statuses to get married, have children, and participate in life to the same extent that other couples do.

In The Community

HIV/AIDS is a global health problem; it is one of the most difficult and unique health crises that human beings have ever faced. Since the beginning of history there have always been *endemic* diseases, and even *epidemics*, such as the Plague, smallpox, cholera, polio, and malaria, but never before has there been a disease that was so widespread and devastating to the entire global community. Every person on the planet has the potential to be affected by HIV, whether it is by personal exposure, the illness or death of a friend or loved one, or the illness of a *role model* in the media. Many people become passionate about HIV/AIDS education after they are diagnosed with the virus, but you can help spread knowledge of HIV/AIDS no matter what your HIV status. You can support the global HIV/AIDS community in many ways: by contributing money or volunteering your time to an HIV/AIDS support organization, by educating yourself, by participating in World AIDS Day events, by talking to your siblings and friends about HIV/AIDS, or even by getting tested for HIV. Disclose your HIV status, negative or positive, to all of your sexual partners, and encourage discussion among your peers about the realities of HIV/AIDS.

Ask the Doctor

My mom was recently diagnosed with HIV. She has been very irritable lately, and doesn't seem to want my help with anything. I don't know if she's taking her medication, and she gets angry with me when I ask about it. I feel so terrible! Is there anything I can do?

Right now, your mother is going through a very difficult time, and she may need time to get used to her diagnosis. She may be angry or sad, but she might not want to talk to you about it. Let her know that you're there for her, but it might be a good idea for you to pull back for a little while to let her get back on her feet.

Real People

Jonathan Larson was an aspiring young composer in New York City in the early 1990s. He had just graduated from college and was working as a waiter to support himself, but his real dream was to write musicals. Inspired by Puccini's La Boheme and several of his close friends' struggles with HIV/AIDS, Jonathan began writing songs. For seven years, he worked on his piece, writing about art, life, and death in the midst of the AIDS crises in the gritty East Village of New York City. On January 25th, 1996, the night after the final dress rehearsal of his show, he collapsed in his apartment and died of an aortic aneurysm. Knowing that he would want his show to go on, his family decided to let the musical play the next day. Little did anyone know, RENT would become a cultural phenomenon: a picture of young people living with—not dying from—AIDS, RENT inspired an entire generation not only to embrace art, but also to understand the great humanity and dignity of those who have lived with AIDS.

(From www.pbs.org/wnet/broadway/stars/larson_j.html)

STRAIGHT FROM THE SOURCE

(From unaids.com, "Human Rights and HIV")

The risk of HIV infection and its impact feeds on violations of human rights, including discrimination against women and marginalized groups such as sex workers, people who inject drugs and men who have sex with men. HIV also frequently begets human rights violations such as further discrimination and violence. Over the past decade the critical need for strengthening human rights to effectively respond to the epidemic and deal with its effects has become evermore clear. Protecting human rights and promoting public health are mutually reinforcing.

Several countries still have policies that interfere with the accessibility and effectiveness of HIV-related measures for prevention and care. Examples include laws criminalizing consensual sex between men, prohibiting condom and needle access for prisoners, and using residency status to restrict access to prevention and treatment services. At the same time, laws and regulations protecting people with HIV from discrimination are not enacted, or fully implemented or enforced.

Reforming laws and policies that are based in deeply-rooted social attitudes and norms such as gender inequality requires multisectoral collaboration. Although not sufficient to change social attitudes, legislation is important for addressing acts of discrimination. Civil society, including organizations of people living with HIV, as well as other parts of society, including police and justice systems, have a critical role to play. International organizations and donors can also play a positive role in support of local and national actors.

The protection of human rights, both of those vulnerable to infection and those already infected, is not only right, but also produces positive public health results against HIV. In particular, it has also become increasingly clear that:

• National and local responses will not work without the full engagement and participation of those affected by HIV, particularly people living with HIV.

• The human rights of women, young people and children must be protected if they are to avoid infection and withstand the impact of HIV.

• The human rights of marginalized groups (sex workers, people who use drugs, men who have sex with men, prisoners) must also be respected and fulfilled for the response to HIV to be effective.

• Supportive frameworks of policy and law are essential to effective HIV responses.

UNAIDS works to help enable States to meet their human rights obligations, and to empower individuals and communities to claim their rights in the context of the HIV epidemic.

What Do You Think?

• Why are human rights an issue when it comes to HIV/AIDS?

• From everything that you've learned, do you think that HIV/AIDS patients should have the same rights as other people?

• How do you think advancing human rights issues might help prevent the spread of HIV/AIDS?

Find Out More

To find out more about what you can do to get involved in the fight against AIDS, check out these Web sites:

www.unaids.org/en/

www.gmhc.org/

www.amfar.org/cgi-bin/iowa/index.html

For More Information on HIV/AIDS

Books

Flanagan, Wendy. *I Am HIV-Positive*. Portsmouth, N.H.: Heinemann, 2003.

Gallant, Joel. 100 *Questions and Answers About HIV and AIDS*. New York: Jones & Bartlett, 2007.

Hinds, Maurene J. *Fighting the AIDS and HIV Epidemic: A Global Battle*. Berkeley Heights, N.J.: Enslow, 2007.

McFarlane, Katerine. *AIDS: Perspectives*. New York: Greenhaven, 2007.

McIntosh, Kenneth. *Living with the Diagnosis: Youth with HIV/AIDS*. Philadelphia: Mason Crest, 2007.

Stine, Gerald. *AIDS Update 2008*. New York: McGraw-Hill, 2008.

Wagner, Viqi. *AIDS: Opposing Viewpoints*. New York: Greenhaven, 2007.

Whiteside, Alan. *HIV/AIDS: A Very Short Introduction*. New York: Oxford University Press, 2008.

Web Sites

AEGIS (AIDS Educational Global Information System)
www.aegis.com

AIDS Info from the U.S. Department of Health and Human Services
www.aidsinfo.nih.gov

AIDSMAP
www.aidsmap.com

AVERT
www.avert.org/aids.htm

The Body: The Complete HIV/AIDS Resource
www.thebody.com

CDC HIV/AIDS Factsheets
www.cdc.gov/hiv/resources/factsheets

HIV InSite (online textbook from the University of
California)
hivinsite.ucsf.edu/InSite

Kaiser Family Foundation Daily HIV/AIDS Report
www.kff.org/hivaids/

Kids' Health: HIV and AIDS
www.kidshealth.com/teen/sexual_health/stds/std_hiv.
html

Mayo Clinic HIV/AIDS
www.mayoclinic.com/health/hiv-aids/DS00005

Medical News Today: HIV & AIDS
www.medicalnewstoday.com/sections/hiv-aids

MedlinePlus
www.medlineplus.gove

Tufts School of Medicine, Nutrition and AIDS
www.tufts.edu/med/nutrition-infection/hiv/

United Nations Development Programme on HIV/
AIDS
www.undp.org/hiv

WHO and AIDS
www.who.int/hiv/en

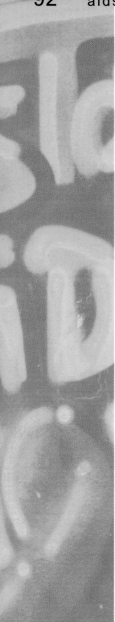

Glossary of HIV/AIDS–Related Terms

When you're reading about HIV/AIDS—or if some-one you know has this disease—you may encounter lots of unfamiliar medical terms. This glossary can help you better understand this complicated disease and its treatments.

Acquired Immunity
The body's ability to fight a specific infection, which can be acquired by having and recovering from an infection, by being vaccinated against an infection, or by receiving antibodies through breast milk.

Acquired Immunodeficiency Syndrome (AIDS)
A disease of the body's immune system caused by HIV (human immunodeficiency virus) that leaves the body vulnerable to life-threatening conditions such as infections and cancer.

Acute HIV Infection
The period of rapid growth of the virus during the two to four weeks after HIV infection. Some (but not all) people will experience flu-like symptoms during this period, which can include fever, sore throat, inflamed lymph nodes, and a rash, lasting from a few days to a few weeks.

AIDS-Defining Condition
Any of a list of 26 illnesses that lead to a diagnosis of AIDS when occurring in a person with HIV. Included in the list are Kaposi's sarcoma, pneumocystis, recurrent pneumonia, pulmonary tuberculosis, invasive cervical cancer, and wasting syndrome.

AIDS-Related Cancer
One of the several cancers that are more common or more aggressive in people with HIV, including lymphomas, Kaposi's sarcoma, and cancers that affect the anus and the cervix.

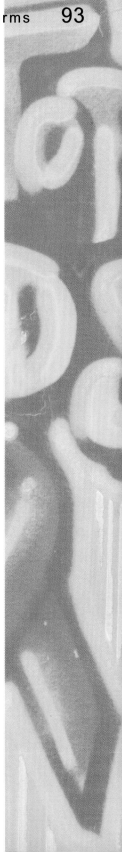

AIDS-Related Complex
A group of conditions that often occur during the early stage of HIV infection, which can include recurrent fevers, unexplained weight loss, diarrhea, herpes, swollen lymph nodes, or fungal infection in the mouth and throat.

Antibody
Also known as immunoglobulin, a protein produced by the body's immune system that recognizes and fights germs and other foreign substances that enter the body.

Antigen
Anything that stimulates the body to produce antibodies to fight it, including bacteria, viruses, and pollen.

Antiretroviral
A medicine that interferes with the ability of a retrovirus (such as HIV) to make more copies of itself.

B-Cell Lymphoma
A type of cancer in the lymphatic tissue, to which people with HIV are more prone.

B Lymphocytes
Also known as B cells, these infection-fighting white blood cells develop in the bone marrow and spleen; in people with HIV, B lymphocytes' ability to do their job is damaged.

Branched Chain DNA Assay (bDNA Assay)
A test that measures a person's viral load (level of HIV present in the blood) to diagnose HIV and monitor disease progression, as well as treatment effectiveness.

Candidiasis
An infection caused by a yeast-like fungus that produces white patches on the skin, nails, and mucus membranes. It is considered an AIDS-defining condition in people with HIV.

Cardiomyopathy

A condition that weakens the heart muscle, which can cause irregular heartbeat and decreased heart function. It may occur in people with HIV.

CD4 Cell

Also known as helper T cell, these infection-fighting white blood cells signal the other cells in the immune system to do their jobs. The number of CD4 cells in a blood sample indicates how healthy the person's immune system is. HIV infects and kills CD4 cells.

CD4 Cell Count

Measuring the number of CD4 cells in a blood sample is one of the most useful ways to tell how far HIV/AIDS has progressed. Health-care providers use this count to determine when to begin or stop therapies and to measure response to treatments. A normal CD4 cell count is between 500 and 1,400 cells per cubic millimeter of blood. When an individual with HIV has a CD4 cell count at or below 200, he is considered to have AIDS.

CD8 Cell

Also called killer T cell, this is a type of white blood cell that is able to recognize and kill cells that are infected by a foreign invader.

Cervical Cancer

A condition in which a cancerous growth forms on the lower portion of the uterus, which is called the cervix; it is a type of cancer to which people with HIV/AIDS are more susceptible.

CIPRA (Comprehensive International Program on Research on AIDS)

A program run by the U.S. NIAID (National Institute on Allergy and Infectious Diseases) to support research and affordable treatment of HIV/AIDS in poor countries.

CMV (cytomegalovirus)
An infectious eye disease that is the most common cause of blindness in people with HIV.

Co-Infection
Infection with more than one germ at a time; for example, a person with HIV may also be infected with hepatitis C or tuberculosis (TB).

Combination Therapy
When two or more drugs are used together to treat HIV, which has proven to be more effective than using a single drug.

Contagious
When a disease passes easily between people through normal day-to-day contact. HIV is not contagious.

Cryptoccosis
An infection caused by a fungus that enters the body through the lungs and usually spreads to the brain. It is considered an AIDS-defining condition in people with HIV.

DNA (deoxyribonucleic acid)
Chemical structure that contains the genetic instructions for reproduction within all cells.

ELISA (enzyme-linked immunosorbent assay)
A sensitive laboratory test used to determine the presence of antibodies to HIV in the blood or saliva. Positive ELISA results should always be confirmed with another test called a Western blot.

End-Stage Disease
The final phase in the course of a disease that will lead to the person's death.

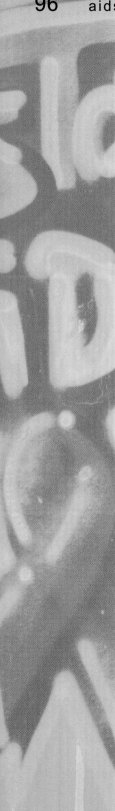

Entry Inhibitors

A class of anti-HIV drugs designed to interfere with HIV's ability to enter a host cell through the cell's surface.

Envelope

The outer protective membrane of HIV cells. Proteins in the envelope allow HIV to attach to and enter host cells.

Enzyme

A protein in the body that helps a chemical reaction happen.

Fusion Inhibitors

A class of anti-HIV drugs that gets in the way of HIV's outer envelope fusing with a host cell's membrane, thus preventing infection of the cell.

GART (genotypic antiretroviral resistance test) or Genotypic Assay

A test that determines if HIV is resistant to a particular drug. The test uses a blood sample to see if any genetic mutations are present that are associated with resistance to specific drugs.

HAART (highly active antiretroviral therapy)

Treatment regimens that aggressively suppress HIV from copying itself and thus slow the progression of HIV disease. It usually combines three or more anti-HIV drugs.

Helper T Cells
See **CD4 Cell**

Hemophilia

A hereditary blood defect, occurring almost exclusively in males, characterized by delayed clotting, which can lead to uncontrolled bleeding, even after minor cuts. Because hemophiliacs often receive blood transfusions to treat injuries, they were exposed to HIV during the 1970s, before doctors realized that the blood supply was infected.

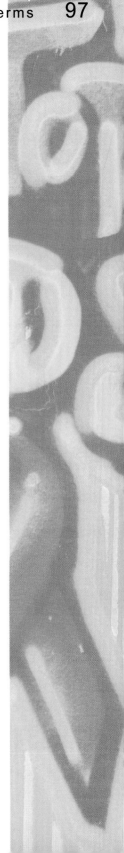

HIV (human immunodeficiency virus)
The virus that causes AIDS.

HIV-1
The type of HIV responsible for most of the HIV infections around the world.

HIV-2
A virus that is closely related to HIV-1, which also causes AIDS. Although the two viruses are very similar, immunodeficiency seems to develop more slowly and to be milder in people who have HIV-2. Most people who have HIV-2 live in West Africa. Drugs used to treat HIV-1 are not always effective against HIV-2.

Immune Response
The body's reaction to a foreign invader, such as a bacteria, virus, or fungus.

Immune System
The cells and organs in the body, including the thymus, spleen, lymph nodes, B and T cells, and antigen-presenting cells, whose job is to protect the body against foreign invaders.

Immunocompromised
Unable to mount a normal immune response because of a damaged immune system.

Immunodeficiency
Unable to produce normal amounts of antibodies and/or immune cells.

Immunoglobulin (IG)
See **Antibody**.

Immunosuppression
Inability of the immune system to function normally (which can be caused by treatments such as chemotherapy or by certain diseases such as HIV).

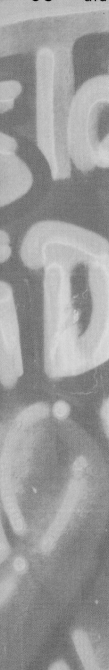

Immunotherapy
Treatment to stimulate or restore the body's ability to fight off diseases.

Incubation Period
The time between when a germ enters the body and when the person develops symptoms.

Infectious
Capable of causing infection.

Integrase
An HIV protein that inserts the virus genetic information into the infected cell.

Integrase Inhibitors
A class of anti-HIV drugs that prevents the integrase protein from inserting genetic information into the host cell.

Integration
The process by which HIV integrase inserts the virus' genetic material into a host cell.

Interleukin-2 (IL-2)
A protein that helps regulate the immune system by increasing the production of certain disease-fighting white blood cells. HIV infection reduces IL-2 levels, but a man-made version of IL-2 is being researched as a way to treat people with HIV.

Interleukin-7 (IL-7)
Another protein that regulates the immune system by increasing the body's production of certain white blood cells. Man-made IL-7 is used to treat HIV because it makes HIV copy itself in infected cells that are resting, allowing anti-retroviral drugs to target HIV in those cells.

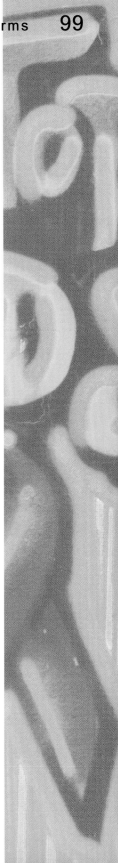

Investigational Drug
Also known as an experimental drug, these medicines' safety and effectiveness have not yet been thoroughly tested.

Kaposi's Sarcoma (KS)
A type of cancer caused by an overgrowth of blood vessels, causing pinkish-purple bumps or spots on the skin. These can also occur inside the body, especially in the intestines, lungs, and lymph nodes, and when this happens, the condition can become life-threatening. KS is considered an AIDS-defining condition. A virus called Kaposi's sarcoma herpesvirus (KSHV) or human herpesvirus 8 often accompanies Kaposi's sarcoma.

Killer T Cell
See **CD8 Cell**.

Latency
The time during which an infection is present within the body without producing any noticeable symptoms. Latency may last for a few years with an HIV infection.

Lentivirus
In Latin, *lente* means "slow;" these are viruses that have a long latency period (like HIV).

Lesion
An area on the skin where the tissue is abnormal, such as a sore or an infected patch.

Leukocytosis
An abnormally high white blood cell count, a condition that usually occurs during an infection.

Leukopenia
A lower than normal white blood cell count.

Long-Term Nonprogressors
People who have been infected with HIV for at least 7 years with no symptoms, stable CD4 counts of 600 or more, and no HIV-related diseases.

Lymph
A clear, yellowish fluid that carries white blood cells (which fight disease) from the blood to body tissues.

Lymph Nodes
Small immune system organs that are located throughout the body, where lymph is filtered as it carries white blood cells back from the body tissues to the blood.

Lymphadenopathy Syndrome (LAS)
Swollen and sometimes sore lymph nodes caused by infections (such as HIV, the flu, or mononucleosis) or lymphoma (cancer of the lymph tissue).

Lymphocyte
A type of infection-fighting white blood cell found in the blood and lymph.

Lymphoid Interstitial Pneumonitis (LIP)
A hardening of the parts of the lung that absorb oxygen for which there is no clear treatment. LIP is an AIDS-defining condition in children with HIV.

Lymphokines
Chemical messengers secreted by white blood cells that affect the immune response.

Macrophage
A type of disease-fighting white blood cell that destroys invaders and helps other immune system cells to do their jobs.

Malabsorption Syndrome
When the intestines cannot adequately absorb nutrients. This is a condition that is associated with HIV

that can lead to loss of appetite, muscle pain, and weight loss.

Memory T Cells
A type of infection-fighting T cell that recognizes foreign invaders it has encountered before (either during an earlier infection or from a vaccination). Memory T cells do their jobs faster and more strongly the second time they see the invader.

Meningitis
Inflammation of the membranes around the brain or spinal cord, which can be caused by bacteria, fungus, or a viral infection like HIV.

Microbes
Living organisms that can only be seen through a microscope, including bacteria, protozoa, viruses, and fungi.

Microsporidiosis
An intestinal infection caused by a parasite that causes diarrhea and loss of weight and strength in people with HIV.

Molluscum Contagiosum
A disease of the skin and mucus membranes that causes white or flesh-colored bumps on the face, neck, hands, underarms, and genitals. A virus causes the condition, but in people with HIV, it usually gets worse with time and does not respond to treatment.

Mucocutaneous
Relating to the mucus membranes and the skin (the eyes, mouth, lips, vagina, and anus, for example).

Mutation
A change or adaptation that can be passed down to future generations. The virus that causes AIDS mutates, which means that an individual strain of HIV can adapt to infect

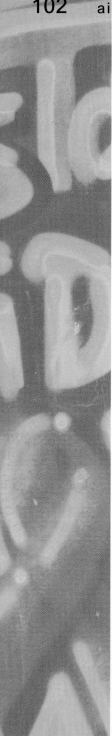

different cell types or to resist certain anti-HIV drugs. Mutations can only occur when the virus is copying itself and not when anti-HIV drugs have suppressed the virus to the point where it is not detectable.

Mycobacterium Avium Complex (MAC)

A life-threatening infection caused by two bacteria found in soil and dust, which is extremely rare in people who do not have HIV. It is considered an AIDS-defining condition in people with HIV.

Myelosuppression

Decreased bone marrow function that means that fewer red blood cells, white blood cells, and platelets (the part of the blood that causes clotting) are produced. It is a side effect of some anti-HIV drugs.

Myopathy

A disease of muscle tissue that can be a side effect of some anti-HIV drugs; HIV itself can also cause it.

Natural Killer Cells (NK cells)

White blood cells that kill tumor cells and other cells infected with viruses or other foreign invaders.

Neuropathy

A disorder caused by damaged nerve cells, which can produce a range of symptoms from a tingly feeling in the toes and fingers to paralysis. Some anti-HIV drugs cause neuropathy, as does HIV itself in some cases.

Neutropenia

A lower than normal number of **neutrophils** in the blood, which can increase the chance of getting bacterial infections. It can be caused by HIV infection, but some anti-HIV drugs also cause it.

Neutrophil

A type of white blood cell that engulfs and kills invaders such as bacteria.

Non-Nucleoside Reverse Transcriptase Inhibitors (NNRTIs)

A kind of anti-HIV drug that binds to and disables the protein that HIV-1 needs to copy itself, bringing an end to HIV-1 multiplication.

Nucleoside

An early version of a nucleotide, the building block that contains DNA and RNA, which are the chemical structures that store the cell's genetic material. Nucleosides must be changed chemically before they can make DNA and RNA.

Nucleoside Analogue Reverse Transcriptase Inhibitor (nuke)

A kind of anti-HIV drug that provides a "bad" version of the building block necessary for HIV reproduction. When it's used instead of a normal nucleoside, reproduction of the virus is halted.

Nucleotide

A building block of the chemical structures (DNA and RNA) that store genetic information within the cell.

Nucleotide Analogue Reverse Transcriptase Inhibitor (nuke)

A kind of anti-HIV drug that provides a "bad" version of a nucleotide, which halts HIV reproduction.

Nukes

See **Nucleoside Analogue Reverse Transcriptase Inhibitor** and **Nucleotide Analogue Reverse Transcriptase Inhibitor**.

Opportunistic Infections (OIs)

Illnesses that occur in people with weakened immune systems, including people with HIV/AIDS. Common OIs in people with AIDS include Pneumocystis carinii pneumonia, histoplasmosis, toxoplasmosis, cryptosporidiosis, and some types of cancers.

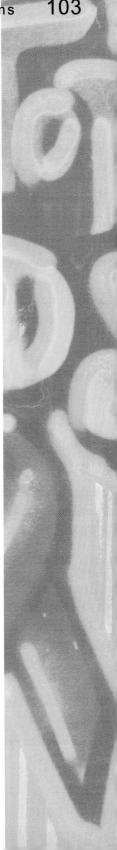

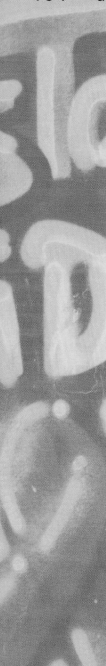

Oral Hairy Leukoplakia (OHL)

A white, hairy, or bumpy patch caused by the Epstein-Barr virus (a member of the herpesvirus family) that appears on the side of the tongue and inside the cheeks, mainly in people with weakened immune systems (including people with HIV).

Osteoporosis

Loss of bone mass, density, and strength, which is usually brought on by old age but can also occur as a result of HIV infection or as a side effect of some anti-HIV drugs.

p24

The protein that surrounds the HIV core where the genetic material is found.

Palliative Care

Medical care that offers no cure but helps reduce the suffering and discomfort caused by the disease's symptoms.

Pancytopenia

A lower than normal level of all types of blood cells, including red blood cells, white blood cells, and platelets.

Paresthesia

Burning, tingling, or pins-and-needles sensations that can be caused as part of neuropathy brought on by certain anti-HIV drugs.

Passive Immunotherapy

A treatment approach that transfers antibodies from one person to another to help the receiver fight infections. An example in HIV treatment is when plasma from healthy HIV-infected people (who have high CD4 counts and high levels of anti-HIV antibodies) is given to people with AIDS who have lost CD4 cells and can no longer make their own antibodies. This treatment has not been very successful with adults, but it is still sometimes used with children who have HIV.

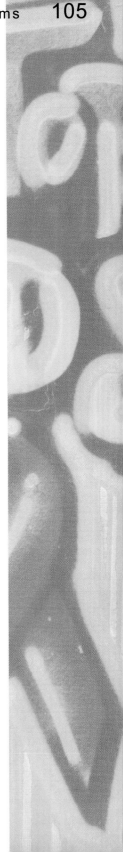

Perinatal Transmission
When a mother with HIV gives her child the virus, either within the womb, during labor and delivery, or through breastfeeding.

Photosensitivity
When skin responds more quickly to sunlight and ultraviolet light, causing sunburns and skin cancer more easily. It can be a side effect of some drugs and can also be caused by HIV infection.

Pill Burden
The number of pills taken each day. A high pill burden may make the person less likely to follow the treatment she needs.

Plasma
The clear, liquid part of the blood in which red blood cells, white blood cells, platelets, nutrients, and wastes are suspended.

Pneumocystis Jiroveci Pneumonia (PCP)
A lung infection that occurs in people with weakened immune systems, including those with HIV, whose first symptoms are difficulty breathing, high fever, and a dry cough. It is considered an AIDS-defining condition in people with HIV.

Post-Exposure Prophylaxis (PEP)
Administration of anti-HIV drugs within 72 hours of a high-risk exposure (such as unprotected sex, needle sharing, or injury) to help prevent HIV infection.

Protease
An enzyme that breaks down proteins into smaller chunks.

Protease Inhibitors (PIs)
A kind of anti-HIV drug that prevents HIV from reproducing by disabling HIV protease.

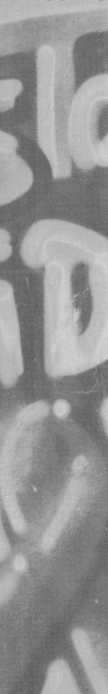

Protease-Sparing Regimen
An anti-HIV drug regimen that does not include a PI.

Protozoa
Tiny, one-celled animals that cause diseases, especially in people with weakened immune systems (including those with HIV). AIDS-defining infections such as toxoplasmosis and cryptosporidiosis are caused by protozoa.

Pulmonary
Having to do with the lungs.

q.d.
Once a day dosing instructions.

q.i.d.
Four times a day dosing instructions.

R5-Tropic Virus
A strain of HIV, also called M-tropic virus.

Receptor
A protein on the surface of a cell that acts as a binding site for substances outside the cell (such as HIV).

Remission
The time during which symptoms diminish or disappear, although the person is still infected.

Retrovirus
A type of virus that stores its genetic information in a single-strand RNA molecule, then builds a double-strand DNA version using an enzyme called reverse transcriptase, which is then integrated into the host cell's own genetic material. HIV is a retrovirus.

Reverse Transcriptase (RT)
An enzyme found in HIV and other retroviruses that converts single-strand RNA into double-strand DNA.

RNA (ribonucleic acid)
The chemical structure that carries genetic instructions for some viruses.

Seborrheic Dermatitis
A skin condition common in people with HIV where the skin is covered with loose, greasy, or dry scales that are white or yellowish. It can occur on the scalp, eyelids, eyebrows, ears, lips, and along any skin folds.

Sepsis
A blood-borne infection, usually caused by bacteria, to which people with HIV are more prone.

Superinfection
A new infection on top of an existing infection, such as when a person with HIV-1 becomes infected with a new strain of HIV. Superinfection makes treatment more challenging.

T Cell
A type of disease-fighting white blood cell, which includes CD4 and CD8 cells. The "T" stands for thymus, where T cells mature.

Therapeutic HIV Vaccine
A vaccine used to treat a person who is already infected with HIV to boost his immune response and better control the virus.

Thymus
An organ behind the breastbone in the chest where infection-fighting T cells develop.

t.i.d.
Three times a day dosing instructions.

Tolerability
How well a medicine can be tolerated—or endured—by a person taking it.

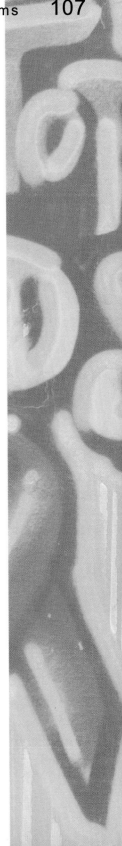

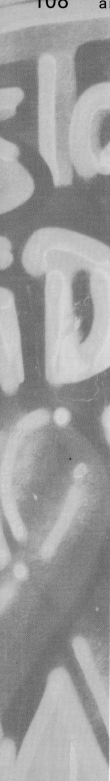

Tolerance
A decreased response to repeated doses of a drug.

Toxoplasmosis
An infection caused by a protozoa that is carried by cats and birds, and is also found in soil contaminated by cat feces and in pork. Toxoplasmosis is an AIDS-defining condition in people with HIV.

Transcription
The step in the HIV life cycle when its DNA is used as a template to create copies of its RNA.

Translation
The step that follows transcription, where the genetic information in the RNA is used to build new copies of HIV.

Vaccine
A substance that stimulates the body's immune response to prevent or control an infection. Researchers are testing vaccines both to prevent and treat HIV/AIDS, but there is currently no approved vaccine.

Viral Load
The amount of HIV RNA in a blood sample, which is an important indicator of the disease's progression.

Virus
A microscopic organism that requires a host cell in order to make more copies of itself. The cold and the flu are both caused by a virus—and so is AIDS.

Western Blot Test
A laboratory technique used to detect HIV proteins in the blood, which is used to confirm a positive ELISA.

Bibliography

"Avert.org: Averting AIDS and HIV" www.avert.org (Accessed May 12, 2008)

Department of Health and Human Services "HIV and Its Treatment: What you Should Know" www.aidsinfo.hhs. gov (Accessed May 12, 2008)

"Benefits of Antiretroviral Drugs" www.aidstruth.org/ new/science/arvs(Accessed May 22 2008)

NGOs International HIV/AIDS Alliance www.aidsalliance.org/sw7119.asp (Accessed May 13, 2008)

Act UP "Aids Cure Project" www.actupny.org/ACP/ ACPQ%26A.html Accessed May 14 2008

Wagner, Wynn "Day One" www.aegis.org/topics/dayone Accessed May 13 2008

"Exposure" www.aegis.org/exposure Accessed May 12 2008

BBC "Have Your Say: AIDS Drugs" news.bbc.co.uk/1/ hi/talking_point/3247391.stm

The Safeguards Project "Safer the Better: My Story"www. safeguards.org/?p=73 Accessed May 13 2008

Food and Drug Adminstration (USA) "HIV and AIDS: Medicines to Help You" www.fda.gov/womens/medi-cinecharts/hiv.htmlAccessed May 12 2008

World Health Organization "HIV and AIDS" www.who. int/topics/hiv_aids/en/

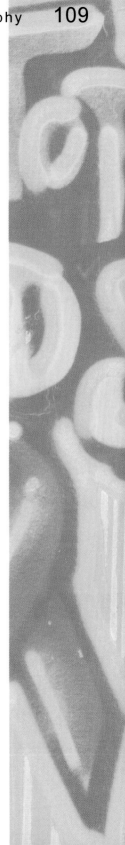

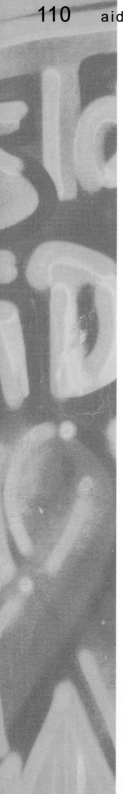

American Pyschological Association "Office on AIDS: Teaching Tip Sheets" www.apa.org/pi/aids/teachtip. htmlAccessed May 12 2008

National Institutes of Allergy and Infectious Diseases " AIDS Vaccines" www3.niaid.nih.gov/research/topics/ HIV/vaccines/ Accessed May 14 2008

American Medical Association "Access to Sterile Syringes" www.ama-assn.org/ama/pub/category/1808. htmlAccessed May 12 2008

"FDA HIV/AIDS Time Line" www.fda.gov/oashi/aids/ miles.html Accessed May 13, 2008

World Health Organization "Condom Facts and Figures" www.wpro.who.int/media_centre/fact_sheets/ fs_200308_Condoms.htm Accessed May 14 2008

Index

Picture Credits

Dreamstime.com
   Kuzma, p. 55
   Mark_lorch, p. 45
   Ricklordphotography, p. 41
   Romkaz, p. 46
   Sebcz, p. 27, 76
   Vadkoz , p. 69

iStock.com
   Kaliciak, Jan, p. 71
   Paternoster, Marcos, p. 36

Ranplett, p. 35

Jupiterimages
pp: 28–29, 33, 42, 83, 48, 57, 60

National Cancer Institute
Nicholson, Trudy, p. 74

To the best knowledge of the publisher, all other images are in the public domain. If any image has been inadvertently uncredited, please notify Harding House Publishing Service, Vestal, New York 13850, so that rectification can be made for future printings.

About the Author

C.E. Boberg lives in Ohio and Seattle, Washington. She has experience with emergency and wilderness medicine and is currently furthering her education in chemistry.

About the Consultant

Elise DeVore Berlan, MD, MPH, FAAP, is a faculty member of the Division of Adolescent Health at Nationwide Children's Hospital and an Assistant Professor of Clinical Pediatrics at The Ohio State University College of Medicine. She completed her Fellowship in Adolescent Medicine at Children's Hospital Boston and obtained a Master's Degree in Public Health at the Harvard School of Public Health. Dr. Berlan completed her residency in pediatrics at the Children's Hospital of Philadelphia, where she also served an additional year as Chief Resident. She received her medical degree from the University of Iowa College of Medicine. Dr. Berlan is board certified in Pediatrics and board eligible in Adolescent Medicine. She provides primary care and consultative services in the area of Young Women's Health, including gynecological problems, concerns about puberty, reproductive health services, and reproductive endocrine disorders.